# Hello Susan, It's Me, Cancer!

## How to LIVE Without Chemotherapy, Radiation or Hormone Treatments

**Susan D'Agostino**

Hello Susan, It's Me Cancer!

Copyright © 2013 by Susan D'Agostino

ISBN: 978-1-927559-05-5
www.healingeverybody.com

Promontory Press
www.promontorypress.com

First Revised Edition: April 2013

Cover by CP Design

Printed in Canada

0 9 8 7 6 5 4 3 2 1

# Disclaimer

This book is to be used alongside your own guidance and healing advisors. No two paths to healing are the same and results may vary. Be willing to take responsibility for your own health and healing and use all that resonates with you. Nothing contained in this book is meant to replace the advice of health care professionals. This book is not to be used as personal medical advice for any one person. Consult your own health care practitioner. Doing anything recommended or suggested in this book must be done at your own risk. The author has no medical training. This book is the author's personal experience.

# Dedication

*This book is dedicated to Jake and Molly and to all women and men, my sisters and brothers, who keep faith and hope open to possibility.*

# Table of Contents

# Hello Susan,
# It's Me,
# Cancer!

# Introduction

Growing up, I always did my very best, and still somehow felt that I was not good enough. At school, being an average student, I stayed out of trouble, didn't go to house parties and certainly wasn't in the "cool" group. I had many friends though, from the kids who went to the smoke hole at lunchtime to the more studious ones who took school seriously and got good grades. I loved my very best friends the most, the friends I could talk to about all my dreams and disappointments.

I fought depression in my teenage years but I didn't know what it was at the time. A deep sadness came and went throughout my growing up and I had a negative attitude that never left me. I didn't know how *not* to feel negative. Having my own horse as a teenager allowed me some respite. Riding, I could look on the brighter side of things now and then. I rode after school almost daily when my chores were done. I loved to be outdoors. During those times I would let my mind wonder and dream about how I wanted my life to be and how I would be so happy one day.

What really held my interest and fascination was the question of what happened to us when we died. Where did we go? I tried to find books that would tell me the answer but the school library's collection, my only resource, was limited. Slowly, as the years went by, I found more books on the subject and learned we have souls that live on and we don't die at all. Only the body dies.

I read books on dreams and their meanings and progressed to books about psychic teachings, intuition, our sixth sense, our mind and how powerful it is. I loved to read and learn about the astrological signs, handwriting analysis, and I had an insatiable appetite for metaphysics. I knew I had psychic abilities. It had been confirmed many times by known psychics. For years odd things happened to me. I didn't know what they meant or how to figure them out, but I continued to study and read. It was all so amazing and intriguing to me. It was the one thing that held my interest for long periods of time.

I was also interested in nutrition. After graduating from high school I competed a few times in bodybuilding contests and once took third place. I studied what the body needs to be healthy. Eating healthily was, and still is, important to me and I believe we all can improve in this area of our lives.

I got a job that paid well; that was what I wanted at the time. Even though it wasn't my

dream job, it paid the bills and I was just starting out in life so was thankful to have it. When I
finally realized how much the job didn't suit me,
I felt compelled to stay with it. After all it was a
'good' job, and they weren't easy to find. I felt I
needed to ignore feelings and did so consciously.
I now had a mortgage to pay. Where else would
I get paid that much? So, day after day I shut
myself off to any feelings that came up—I simply
went to work every day. Slowly, year after year, I
ignored more and more of my true feelings, putting a smile on my face as I died inside.

I hadn't yet realized that shutting down
emotions also shuts down the immune system.
Looking back, I knew so little about anything.

When I was diagnosed with breast cancer,
I allowed myself to quit my job of over twenty
years, no matter what I would have to face. I figured that if it came to my job or my life, I would
choose my life.

This book is the naked truth about the steps
I took to heal. It tells of how I learned to follow
my inner guidance, chronologically, factually,
and with no frills. It's about the harsh reality of
surviving an emotional block in my body and
the pain and courage it took to release that block.
It outlines the steps I took, how I felt, and how
and why I healed from the ailment our culture is
terrified of—*Breast Cancer*.

The information in this book is for you who
has been recently diagnosed and/or are looking for an alternative, complementary path to

healing. Whether you have done conventional treatments or not I hope the information is helpful to you in moving forward. I searched for a book like this when I was faced with decisions I didn't know how to make. Then, I couldn't find the information I so desperately needed.

I have learned that this disease is an emotional disease. When we align ourselves with truth, connect with our soul and honour who we are, we heal.

Through this book I am holding my hand out to you, or someone you know, who might consider complementary, natural, and alternative ways of healing from what they call breast cancer. Someone held her hand out to me. My friend's friend's mom, a stranger, a woman I had never met, has become my sister. She pointed toward another way of healing. Now, I want to pay it forward.

When cancer came knocking at my door, I realized I needed to take a look at my life. I had been unhappy for a very long time; on most days my life felt empty. I wanted a new lifestyle, I wanted to find work I loved, to feel good. I wanted a purpose. Little did I know that cancer would lead me to feel joy, peace, happiness and love. My soul had had enough. It spoke to me, loud and clear. I needed to change things in my life that were not happy or joyful.

So my journey begins …

# Chapter 1

# CANCER

## Lean Into the Pain

In 2002 I found a lump in my breast, maybe the size of a pea. I had it checked out by a doctor and was told it was a cyst. At that time the doctor asked me if I wanted to have it aspirated. I declined the offer.

Over the next couple of years I noticed that it had started to grow. The lump was getting larger and at the rate it was growing, it would soon be almost as large as my breast.

In 2005 I made an appointment with a naturopath. Though my problem at the time was fatigue, I mentioned to her that I had a lump in my breast. I explained that it had been checked out years before, that it was only a cyst, and that it had started to grow. In my mind's eye, I envisioned scar tissue growing around the cyst.

After examining the lump, the naturopath advised me to have it checked out again. I reluctantly called a doctor in the area who was taking new patients. I was not a go-to-the-doctor kind of person. I usually went once a year to have my thyroid checked, so I didn't have a regular doctor.

The appointment was in June. The doctor examined the lump. He looked worried and told me that I needed an ultrasound. A few days later, on June 28th, I had it. The doctor also made an appointment for me to see a surgeon the following week.

I was advised to get a mammogram directly after the ultrasound. They could fit me in that same day and although I did not want a mammogram, I felt that maybe the medical staff knew best.

Sitting in the waiting room I remember thinking this was certainly not the way I wanted to spend my one precious day off. The room was cold, the technician's hands were cold, and the machine was cold. The environment was not pleasant, especially having to strip naked from the waist up. Putting my breast on the plate was difficult. It seemed that no one noticed that my breast was still attached to the rest of my body. Not being overly endowed in that area, I found there was only so much I could do to get that breast "out there." I leaned in, was told to "turn a little that way," and then the other plate came down, squeezing my breast to the point of agony. What would happen if the lump burst? The lump was hard and that scared me. We had to go through this procedure a couple of times to get a good picture. I wondered who had invented this barbaric machine that could torture a woman so.

I was also scheduled for a core needle biopsy that same week. The core needle biopsy was a very painful experience as well. I felt as if I had been shot by a nail gun, not once but twice. The first shot was taken very near the lump. The second was shot directly opposite the lump, right through my breast. It hurt! As I struggled to catch my breath, tears sprang from my eyes. The pain was beyond my threshold. I took a few deep breaths and could feel that I was about to faint. I was asked by the doctor who "shot" me if I was all right and if there was someone to drive me home. I had driven myself to this appointment. No one had told me that the procedure would be so excruciating I might not feel comfortable driving myself home. Later on someone told me that this was usually done after some sort of numbing medication administered to the area. Either the medication didn't take effect or there had been none administered.

# Chapter 2

# THE SURGEON & SURGERY

## Cut, Wrapped, and Delivered

My appointment with the surgeon was July 6th. As he read through the papers on his desk, this young man looked kindly at me through his glasses and stated that I definitely had cancer. He continued to explain what the process would be and what I would have to do, but I could not believe what he was telling me. As I sat attentively in the chair next to his desk I felt my heart drop into my belly, my throat was suddenly parched. Up until that moment there had been no doubt in my mind that the lump was *not* cancerous. My mind whirled and I could feel a tear run down my cheek, he gently handed me a tissue as I struggled to comprehend what he was telling me. He scheduled me for surgery July 13th, in just one week, to remove the lump and a quarter of an inch of tissue around it, which would amount to approxi-mately a quarter of my breast. They would also take some lymph nodes to see if the cancer had spread there as well.

It was devastating news, to say the least. My life no longer seemed to be my own anymore. I could feel the anxiety welling up inside me at not being in control of anything. I had very strong fears about getting on the "cancer train" and I did not want to be a part of it. Even though my appointments and follow-ups would be with this younger surgeon, he would not be doing the actual surgery. He was new to the area and just beginning his profession. A surgeon specializing in breast "situations" would do the surgery and I would not even meet him before the procedure. At the time I thought this was a peculiar situation. I could feel my stress level rising because the person I was speaking with was not the person who was going to be cutting off a quarter of my breast.

My naturopath was on maternity leave so I spoke about the upcoming surgery to the naturopath who shared the same office. He prescribed some pre-surgery supplements and I went home to fearfully await the surgery date.

On July 13th I was prepped for surgery. One of the nurses asked me several times if I had taken any aspirin. I had not. I could not figure out why she kept asking me—of course I was sure I hadn't taken any. Apparently she was having problems getting the needle into my vein during the surgical prep procedures. I had asked to meet the surgeon and I did for about fifteen seconds. He was tall, handsome and had a nice manner about him, he said hello to me and shook my hand, just before I went under.

* * *

I woke up in the hospital room. The surgery had been a success, according to my parents and husband. Like that was supposed to make me feel better! I was in pain, my breast was bandaged, I had an auxiliary drain coming out of my rib cage from the lymph node removal, and I was very thirsty. I had brought along some juice so I would have something nutritious when I came out of surgery. I was also very groggy. When two of my close friends came by, my parents and husband went home. One of my dear friends held the provided small pan under my chin while I threw up the juice I had just drunk. The other friend left the room during this incident because she felt nauseated and couldn't tolerate someone throwing up. I definitely couldn't blame her. I felt like a mess, I was in pain, and kept falling asleep.

Later, it was difficult for me to sleep through the night, so I accepted the sleeping pills or pain relievers, whatever it was they offered me. The nurses were very kind. One especially was very understanding, telling me she had been through it twice. I couldn't even imagine … When daylight finally came, my husband arrived to pick me up. I felt horrible, I felt sorry for myself, I was angry at the whole situation, I wanted to go home, I was in pain and I felt dizzy. My arm was in a sling and I had a hose protruding from my side.

Lying on the couch later, I cried. I felt horribly sorry for myself and angry at everything. I hated it all. My husband had begun renovating our home a few months before so everything looked bad, and I felt bad. Since the family room had been torn apart, there was nowhere to rest. The living room was too cold and I felt there was nowhere I could be warm and comfortable.

# Chapter 3

# THE NURSES

## No Pain, No Gain

The following day, a nurse was to come to our home to check on me and change the dressing on the surgery site. I tried to stay in bed as long as I could so I wouldn't have to deal with anything. When she arrived and I answered the door, my dog, Molly, was barking. The nurse had questions for me, and she was very put off by my dog, asking me if I could put her outside. I refused, but told her that if she wanted we could talk upstairs. I apologized for my dog barking but explained that Molly was a part of our family. The nurse wasn't impressed, to say the least, and frankly, I didn't give a damn.

She changed the dressing and told me that it looked good. Maybe it did from her point of view, but from mine, it didn't look so good. The stitches went around the nipple area and continued toward the inner part of my breast. The incision was approximately two inches in

12

length. The inner lower quadrant of my breast was flat. It looked horrible, like it wasn't a part of me anymore. I felt mutilated, as if a piece of me had been carved out of my body. There was also a stitched-up gash under my armpit where they had removed the lymph nodes. The plastic tube protruding from my side, just above my ribs, had a plastic container at its end, which was filling with fluid from the damaged lymph node area. It was pinned to my underwear. I was in pain but refused to take any of the prescribed drugs. I was not about to take any more painkillers. I would deal with the pain as it wasn't all that bad.

After the nurse left I stared numbly at the stitches that held my breast together. My eyes stung with tears. I felt so weak and violated. *Look what they did to me!* I felt branded. And the nurse thought it looked good.

The following day a different nurse came to attend to my dressing. My dog didn't bother her. On the third day a male nurse came to assist me. He asked if I had had a bowel movement since my surgery. "No," I told him, beyond embarrassed. He told me I needed to take a laxative. He explained that the drugs used in surgery cause constipation. *Why hadn't anyone else told me that?* He didn't have any laxatives with him, but advised that it was extremely important to deal with it. He asked me if the other nurses had spoken to me about this issue. They hadn't. He was surprised—usually that was the first question asked. Great, just my luck—no one telling me until three days later!

My dear friend, a pharmacy technician, brought me some natural stool softeners and fortunately, they fixed the problem.

The days passed slowly. The hose still protruded from my side. Bathing was an adventure in itself as I tried to wash my armpit without getting any water onto the hose. My husband tried his best to help me. I couldn't use one arm, so it was really awkward and he wasn't very helpful. He tried his best to wash my hair, but I wasn't used to anyone helping me bathe so it was very frustrating. I took my frustration out on him, I'm afraid, and told him he wasn't doing it right, and how he could do it better—but he just wasn't listening.

I couldn't find any books about alternative and natural ways of healing from breast cancer. All I found were stories of how women had gone through chemotherapy and radiation. I threw the book across my bedroom. *I did not want to be part of it!*

I didn't want to die, but maybe that was what was going to happen. I remembered wanting to die when I was fourteen years old. I remembered wishing I were dead, that I would just disappear. I remembered praying for death, so long ago.

But now, in my bedroom, in pain, I felt angry. I yelled at God through my tears, "Oh no, not now! I made that wish when I was fourteen years old, I wished I could have disappeared, I

14

wished I were dead and I wanted to die. It's too late now, you had your chance, that was thirty years ago, now I want to see how my life turns out!" I finally had my chance to die but now I wanted to live!

I called the doctor's office to find out if they had gotten the results back from the lymph node biopsy. They had not, so I asked them to please telephone me when they did receive them. Hopefully, no news was good news.

The guy who was doing some dry walling for us during this time said cancer was caused by resentment; I needed to "forgive" as the cure. I thought it was an interesting concept.

My arm and surgery area were still very tender and feeling prickly and itchy. I kept my arm bent, my wrist held against my breast; otherwise it felt as if the stitches might pull apart. My arm felt numb, especially the back of my arm and armpit. If I pressed against the outer side of my breast near the armpit, I could feel a sensation in my elbow.

* * *

Over the previous year or so, wherever I went I noticed the numbers 1111 for some reason, whether on the clock or the mileage on my vehicle. I noticed it on a receipt in a book I got from the library. Even once while waiting in line at a checkout, the customer ahead of me was asked his phone number and the last four digits were 1111. I had seen this series of numbers often enough to realize that it must have some meaning. I asked friends if they knew what it meant. Nobody did.

* * *

I was allowed to heal from surgery for a couple of months before I had to think about treatments. A nurse still came to my home every day to change the dressing and to check on the drainage. Twelve days after surgery I had an appointment with the surgeon I had been consulting. He told me that they had removed seven lymph nodes and two were cancerous.

I simply stared at him, stunned, I opened my mouth to speak but no words came through. My mind was having a one sided conversation on its own. *How could this be? Why hadn't my doctor contacted me?* He also said that the surgeon who performed the surgery had said that if I had consulted him pre-surgery, he would have opted to take off my whole breast. My mind was racing as I tried to focus and listen to what he was telling me, but all I could hear was someone speaking far off in the distance saying things I couldn't hear because my heart was pounding so loudly in my ears.

The doctor went on to inform me that I had invasive high-grade ductal carcinoma, grade II, progesterone and estrogen positive. The firm white tumor mass measured 2.7 cm from lateral to medial, 2.6 cm from superior to inferior and up to 2.1 cm in thickness. The surgical margins were clear. The surgical site was healing well, and he recommended that I receive chemotherapy and radiotherapy and, hormone therapy. He would advise the Cancer Agency on my behalf. My husband was with me, and as we left the office, I was crying once again. Fear pulled at me from the inside of my body. I couldn't believe it. I felt powerless; I didn't know what I was going to do. I couldn't believe that my doctor's office had not contacted me with my lymph node results. *Why hadn't they told me?* I had specifically asked them to. I felt betrayed. All I could do was cry.

On Sunday, July 31st, the nurse who arrived at my home examined the auxiliary drain and announced that the tube was ready to come out. I felt like jumping for joy. To finally be rid of that pain in my side meant a great day! She also said that she could do it right then and there, so out it came. There were about four inches of hose (to them it was a tube, to me it was a hose) inside my body, right at the top of my rib cage and, unbeknownst to me, the hose was slightly larger on the inside of my body than what I saw on the outside. Searing pain ripped through my side as she pulled out the hose. The tube felt as if it was on fire, as if it had grown to my ribs. For eighteen days that drainage hose had been a part of my body. Maybe it *had* started to attach itself to me! I was grateful that I was sitting down as she quickly pulled the burning hose out of me. I took several very deep breaths, until the seething pain subsided somewhat. It makes me shudder to this day when I remember that searing pain. Yet I was so grateful that the damn hose was out of my body! When the nurse left, I felt like a lost soul, lost in the scary waters of the unknown. *Why was this happening to me? Why did I have to go through this? What did I do to deserve this?* Sometimes self-pity is a good place to be, and I wallowed in it. I comforted myself with self-pity, sadness, and fatigue and I cried for myself.

A couple of days later, as I sat outside on the swing, a hawk flew past me and landed in the neighbour's tree. It sat there for a good long while and I sat and watched it as it sat and watched me. Finally it flew away. I had never seen a hawk so close before that day, nor have I since. To me it meant there was something watching over me. I felt peculiarly safe and guided, even though I had no proof that what I was trusting in was "right."

The symbol of the hawk intrigued me and I looked for an interpretation:

It represents a messenger that shows up in our life as a reminder to pay attention to the subtle messages that show up. Hawks have the skill to be in the real and the unseen realms connecting both worlds together. Seeing the bigger picture allows the hawk to see past, present and future all at the same time. For a person with this totem it symbolizes prophetic insight. A tendency towards thinking too much causes the clear vision to be lost. It reminds us to keep our analytical mind under control and not allow it to run wild.

It indicates that we cannot hide from our destiny. Sooner or later it will catch up with us.

Humankind is to awaken from their spiritual amnesia and align with the original intention of their soul. The hawk suggests we evaluate who we think we are and our self-created illusions so our inner truth may rise within us.

Hawk opens us to higher consciousness and reunites us with Great Spirit. This totem can be bitter sweet. If we accept it we will be asked to surrender to anything that doesn't honor truth.

Later that day a quiet inner voice spoke to me. *This will be the best thing that ever happened to you*, it said. In spite of everything that was happening to me, somewhere in my heart I knew it was true. I felt a welcome feeling of comfort in knowing this.

We lived within walking distance of a beautiful urban forest. I greeted the trees, birds, and everything else that lived there whenever I walked there. Having always loved the outdoors, the feeling was safe and welcoming. I felt good there; this was nature at its finest. Each walk inspired me about life and gave me a sense of freedom. This environment helped the endorphins open my being so that I could communicate with the angels and my guides. In that shady retreat, I received insights and knowledge.

When I was up to it, I went for long walks in the forest with my dog. Friends occasionally joined us but I didn't always feel good. I felt numb emotionally and my right armpit, where they had removed the lymph nodes, felt numb as well. I still couldn't believe this was happening to me. I spoke with friends over the telephone daily. One of my close friends wrote an affirmation for me from the book *The Power of Your Subconscious Mind* by Dr. Joseph Murphy. I read that affirmation every single morning for over six months while I brushed my teeth.

I was never able to memorize the affirmation, for some reason. Maybe because my mind was so full of everything else and I was so stressed out.

A neighbour told me about her daughter-in-law who pursued natural therapies after chemotherapy. While I wondered what she had done, I just wasn't in the right frame of mind or mood to find out more.

I kept copies of all my test results for my own files. When I asked the doctor for them, he agreed to give them to me. After my appointment I wanted to pick them up but the copies weren't ready. I wondered if he really cared whether I received them or not. I was feeling too teary to wait for them, so I left and picked them up at a later time.

I had an appointment at the hospital to get my arm measured by a physiotherapist to ensure that it wasn't swelling from the lymph node removal. I really liked the physiotherapist. She told me about support groups in the area. My arm seemed fine— the measurements were nearly the same as before the surgery. "Always do what you think you should do," was her advice to me.

I thought it was interesting and odd that she said that to me out of the blue. Sometimes we hear things that only later make sense. Maybe this is how divine messages reach us when we need to receive them.

## Chapter 4

# NATUROPATH #1

## Don't Worry About Anything,
## Just Pray About Everything

On August 9th, test results in hand, I went to see a naturopath. In so many words he told me that it looked pretty bad. He mentioned natural treatments, but told me I would have to take many supplements. When I asked if he thought I should do chemotherapy, he told me I should. I got the feeling that my case was serious enough that he did not want to take it on. With my heart in my throat, I drove home.

# Chapter 5

# THE ONCOLOGIST

## Mad Professor

Two days later, on August 11th, I had a two-and-ahalf-hour appointment with an oncologist. The feeling of fear and dread in my chest made it hard to breathe. After my shower that morning, I noticed a bird pecking on the bathroom window. That had never happened before and I wondered if it was some sort of sign. It made me feel very alert and scared.

My husband was to come home from work to drive me to the Cancer Agency (that is what it is called here) for my appointment. Before he arrived, I heard a tapping sound—another little bird was pecking at the kitchen window. It was a chickadee, I found out later. The appearance of chickadees symbolizes *optimism*.

But here and now, seeing the little bird trying to get my attention, I felt frightened and concerned. I could feel the hair standing up on the back of my neck. *What could this possibly mean? Was it that something or someone was trying to get my attention?* The bird would peck on the window, then sit on the ledge and stare at me. I didn't know what this was all about, but it made me feel very peculiar, as if all my senses were somehow magnified. I felt so aware of everything; I could feel my heart pounding and the dread radiating from somewhere deep within. I felt more sensitive to my every thought, my every move, I felt more alert and I was aware of the fear engulfing my being. As we were leaving the house I began to cry and felt extremely anxious. I told my husband I didn't want to go, but he told me that we had to. I felt as if I was being taken to the gas chamber. Fear gripped me until I could hardly breathe. I was living in a nightmare from which, maybe, I would wake up. But no, it just kept going on and on.

When we arrived at the Cancer Agency, everyone was bustling here and there. Everyone had duties to do. I had to fill out a three-page form with the usual details. My writing didn't look like my own; it was larger than normal and I could feel the pressure I was putting on the pen. I thought it was going to go right through the paper. I felt so angry. I did not want to be there. Everyone was nice as pie, too nice as far as I was concerned. It was as though they needed me to like them and I felt that they were faking it, that they weren't being truthful or real. In this time of heightened anxiety and fear, it was as if I could see right through their attempts to make me believe they were good, kind, and likable.

The nurse at the Cancer Agency was very nice, too, way too nice, and spoke to us in her very nice voice. She had me stand on the scale, recorded my weight, and asked me questions. I didn't like her 'nice' manner. I didn't like the Cancer Agency.

I didn't like that it was going to be two and a half hours until I could go home. I didn't want to answer her questions. It just felt all wrong. When the oncologist entered the room, I didn't like him from the start. He had small, beady eyes and a balding head; to me he looked like a soulless, evil doctor. It was his job to figure out what and how many chemotherapy treatments I would receive. His recipe for me was to receive eight chemotherapy treatments using three different drugs. I would finish some time in January. It was now August. So he thought he was going to poison me until January, did he? Well he didn't know that I was not about to be led down that garden path. I was not about to board the 'cancer train.'

After chemotherapy, I would be given radiation treatments. I would stay on hormone therapy, in the form of a pill, for five years. It would push me right through menopause, he told me, almost happily, as though it were a good thing. I "wouldn't have to be bothered by all the symptoms normally associated with menopause." Well I didn't want to be pushed through menopause! I felt I still had a few good years before menopause!

He said he would write a prescription for a wig, and I would then go for some blood tests. He told me they had a new pill that took care of nausea; it actually made patients feel hungry, so I might even gain a few pounds! This guy was really pushing it with me.

Not only would I totally kill off my own immune system, lose my hair, and be sick, but I might also gain a few pounds, suffer radiation burns, and be pushed through menopause.

I was enraged at the whole process. It just did not make any sense to me. I could not wrap my head around this way of thinking. He seemed like a very intellectual type. When I told him that I drank wine and smoked one to five cigarettes a day, he shrugged and gave me a small, rather superior smile. "Do whatever you have to do to get through it," he told me. I expected my husband to ask some questions, but neither of us knew what to ask. I sat in the chair and I tried to listen to what he was saying, but all I heard was *blah, blah, blah*. I was stressed to the maximum.

The oncologist wanted to examine my incisions. He asked my husband if he wanted to stay in the room or step out. My husband opted to step out. Furious and indignant, I snapped at my husband that he would indeed be staying in the room with us! I couldn't believe he would willingly leave me in that room, scared and defenseless, while that man, the oncologist, looked at my breast! I was feeling very vulnerable. The oncologist stepped out while I changed out of my blouse and put on the hospital gown. He came back into the room and looked at my stitchedup breast and commented on how well I was healing and how obviously I took very good care of myself and that I must work out because I had a good, strong, healthy upper body … *Why was he looking at my body?* I had the urge to scream at him, right in his face, that maybe he should just look at whatever he was supposed to be looking at and keep all his damn comments to himself! But I sat there while he examined me, biting my tongue, so as not to reveal how humiliated, scared, and enraged I felt.

He said I was to continue healing. On September 14th I was to attend a teaching class for chemotherapy. I felt so defenseless—a teaching class for chemotherapy. I didn't even want to know what that entailed. On September 15, I would begin chemotherapy.

As we drove home from that experience, I wondered out loud why he had to look at my breast. I was sure he had read the reports from my surgeon that stated I was healing well. The memory of the experience made me shudder and feel slightly violated.

A couple of days later in my journal I wrote:

*My body is screaming NOOO!!!!!!!! No to the morbid chemotherapy!!*

# Chapter 6

# THE BONE SCAN

"Is she going to make it, Bones?"

"Don't know, Jim."

Star Trek

One of my friends told me that her friend's mom, who had had stage IV breast cancer, pursued alternative treatment and was doing well, eight years later. They (the doctors and oncologists) had given her six months to live, yet she was still alive and well. Another lady I knew told me cancer is caused by unresolved issues and an imbalance in the body. She knew a medical intuitive and gave me his card.

According to www.thomas-moore.com:

"A medical intuitive can see the entire energy body. He can also see inside the body just like a full-coloured x-ray. As a medical intuitive, he

28

has the ability to intuit the resonating, debilitating factor in a person's illness. This can be caused by a negative emotion. An intuitive more often than not can connect this emotional cause of their physical ailment or disease. He also has the ability to see a past life which may be causing a problem in the present life."

Another friend borrowed a book for me from her massage therapist. *The Cure for all Cancers*, by Hulda Regehr Clark, Ph.D., ND, gave me insight into what causes cancer and how to eliminate the toxins from my body. It was a very interesting book and it gave me hope that I could heal without chemotherapy treatment, radiation, or hormone drugs. I cleaned out all the poisonous, carcinogenic cleaning products from my home. I stopped using makeup, antiperspirant, and anything else that contained a known carcinogen. I started using soap and shampoo that did not contain any known toxins. It's unbelievable that so many of our toiletries, which we put directly on our skin, contain known cancer-causing ingredients, all of which are government approved. So many people are getting cancer and we cannot figure out why. One would think the government would have caught on by now.

August 15th was my appointment for a bone scan which would determine whether or not cancer had invaded my bones. Once again fear welled up inside my body—what if it had? Maybe I was going to die.

The technician conducting the test told me

that she wasn't allowed to comment one way or the other about what she saw on her screen. I had to lie on a platform that was slowly drawn into a machine—it was extremely claustrophobic. The machine moved very slowly and all I could do was pray. The technician was so kind. Without her 'telling' me one way or the other, I left knowing that my bones were clear. My mind could now rest about that one.

# Chapter 7

# MY FRIEND'S FRIEND'S MOM

## A Little Bird Told Me

I was on a roller coaster of emotions. I wanted to believe there was a natural way to heal from this disease, but I did not know anyone with knowledge of how to begin or what to do. I had only a few weeks until I was supposed to start chemotherapy. My mind was racing most days. I did not know where to begin and I was stressed out, exhausted, and emotional. I felt I was waiting to get sick, or maybe waiting to die. It just didn't make any sense to me to kill off my immune system. What made sense to me was to build my immune system up. But I didn't know how to do that on my own. On a good day, when I considered following the natural way, I felt really good and I had lots of energy. I went for long walks in the forest with my dog. On a bad day, when I didn't feel so good, I felt depressed, hopeless, and thought maybe it was my time to die. Some days I stayed in my pajamas all day; some days I stayed in bed all day.

On a warm Saturday, August 20th, I opted to stay in bed all day; I didn't see a purpose in getting up. A friend telephoned me at 2:30 in the afternoon and asked how I was doing. I was crying and watching TV in bed. She once again told me of her friend's mother who had used natural treatments and wondered, if she got me the telephone number, would I call her friend's mom? I told her the lady would think it was a prank call because I could not speak without crying. She said she would call the lady and have her friend's mom call me. I agreed to that arrangement. After I hung up the telephone, a huge surge of energy filled my body. There was hope! I threw my blanket off and I ran to the bathroom to have a shower. I was so excited and energized—suddenly I felt so good. I showered and then waited for my telephone to ring.

When the phone did ring a while later it was her. I explained to her where I was in the process, that I had had surgery and a partial mastectomy, and she began to speak very passionately about what I needed to do. I told her I smoked a little and I thought she was going to come right through the telephone at me! She told me, very loudly, that I couldn't do both! She told me to just stop it; that smoking cigarettes robs the body of oxygen! Either I keep smoking and do conventional treatments or I don't take one more puff and do natural treatments. She told me about some treatments—coffee enemas, intravenous vitamin C, and drinking freshly squeezed juices—which cleanse the body. She knew of a naturopath who maybe could help me. She told me about an integrated healing clinic in the city, explained that cancer hates oxygen, so exercise is good. She also suggested letting go of the fear since cancer feeds on fear. Stop eating sugar and stop drinking alcohol.

She said to take one day at a time and acquire a passion for life. I honestly didn't have a clue about how to get a passion for life. She directed me to go to the beach and give everything I didn't want back to the universe. She asked me what I could do today. I thought that maybe I could go to the organic vegetable farm and buy some vegetables to juice.

She shared very little about her story. She had gone to Mexico for natural treatments eight years before. At that time, the doctors here had given her only months to live. I have never met this lady in person, but I am eternally grateful for her passion and for helping me to save my life. I never had another cigarette.

After that telephone conversation, I went to the organic farm for some fresh vegetables to juice. Whenever my friends and I walked on the beach we spent time thinking about what we wanted to give back to the universe. We would throw a rock into the ocean as a symbol for everything we wanted to give back. Then we would throw a rock and ask for what we wanted. We threw many rocks into the ocean that summer.

# Chapter 8

# MY DECISION TO USE ALTERNATIVE TREATMENTS

## Go With the Flow

My mind was racing. Should I wait around until I was sick and had no hair and felt crappy after having poisoned my whole system or should I work on improving my immune system and becoming even healthier? I thought about it while sitting on my sofa, walking on the beach, walking through the forest, when I went to bed at night, and when I woke up in the morning. I thought about it day after day after day.

Engulfed by mind-numbing indecision, fear pulled at my insides as I wondered what I should do. *How do I decide? What if I make the wrong choice? What if it is just my time to die? What should I do?* I noticed that when I imagined myself doing the chemotherapy, I felt really down and sad, weepy and weak. When I imagined myself proceeding with alternative therapies and being healthy, I felt myself wanting to move forward. I felt in control, strong, as if I had a purpose, and it felt good.

Finally, alone, sitting on my sofa in the torn-apart, partially renovated family room, I decided to use alternative and natural treatments to strengthen my immune system instead of destroying it. That made total sense to me.

I decided to do whatever I needed to. I had heard that alternative therapies were expensive, so I decided I would have to put all thoughts about how much it was going to cost aside and do what I had to do. I had always been very careful about spending. I realized that I would have to let that go for now so all my energy could be put into healing from this disease they call breast cancer. I made my decision, realizing that not all my friends and family would be in favour of my decision. That was okay, because I was going to trust only myself through this. If people didn't like it, they would have to deal with it on their own. I told my husband first, then my parents, then the rest of my friends and family. Most of them supported my decision, or if they didn't, they didn't say so. One of my dear friends, the pharmacy technician, cried; she was afraid she was going to lose me. I told her that if I did conventional treatments she might lose me, too. Little by little, as time went on, she seemed more accepting of it.

Two of my sisters-in-law suggested natu- ropaths they had heard of by word-of-mouth. I began forming a list. I would search until I found who I was looking for. I was on a mission.

# Chapter 9

# SUPPORT GROUP
## #1

## Never Be Ashamed to Cry

I was given information from the hospital about cancer support groups that met in the area. There were two. One group was cancer in general and they met every third Thursday. The other group was breast cancer only and they met every first and third Monday of the month. I decided to attend one and it happened to be a Thursday. Maybe someone there was going the natural route as well and I could get some information, a name, or some kind of lead for my situation. I felt strong that day, not too weepy. I found the meeting place. The facilitator was very friendly and kind. There were about ten of us sitting around a large table. Most were women older than myself and there was one man around my age. I was introduced to the group as the "new girl." I told everyone that I wanted to do natural and alternative treatments. I wanted to build up my immune system instead of destroying it with chemotherapy, radiation, and pills that might make me gain weight. I could feel the tension in the room as one person stated that it might be better to gain a few pounds than to lose my life. All of a sudden a huge wave of grief came over me and I started to sob, right there in the meeting! I could not get a handle on it and I didn't even have a tissue because I had been feeling fine earlier. Someone handed me a box of tissues and I tried to listen to what everyone was saying but instead I cried. You know – the big, ugly uncontrollable crying thing. It came over me like a tidal wave and all I could do was ride it out. I must have picked up on someone else's energy because I knew this weeping was not from me.

# Chapter 10

# NATUROPATH
## #2, #3, & #4

## Who's Driving the Bus?

I made an appointment with the naturopath my friend's friend's mom had told me about. This naturopath specialized in treating cancer patients. I also joined a yoga class. I eagerly waited for the day of my appointment. When it finally arrived, a friend came with me. When my friend's friend's mom had called to tell me what to do, who to see, and so on, I had taken notes. I was beginning to realize I couldn't remember anything. It seemed as if my mind could not hold any information whatsoever, maybe because I was so incredibly over-stressed and exhausted. So, with my blue coil-back notebook and test results in hand, optimistic attitude, and friend at my side, off I went to see the naturopath.

She looked over my results. As I sat at the edge of the chair eagerly awaiting her comments, she looked at me from across her desk and the words that came out of her mouth floored me. She could not help me. The cancer, invasive high-grade ductal carcinoma, stage II, was progesterone and estrogen positive and she was not comfortable treating me. She did, however, know of someone who might be able to help. She would fax my test results to a naturopath she knew who was on Vancouver Island, a two-and-ahalf-hour ferry ride away.

I kept my composure as my friend and I walked out of the office and then I completely fell apart. The drive home was difficult. I cried and my friend cried. We couldn't believe the naturopath couldn't help me. I was devastated. My solar plexus tightened as the fear invaded my body. I had told many of my friends and family that I was seeing a naturopath who might be able to help me. I felt crushed, as now I had to tell them that she couldn't help me. I also wondered if I would ever find the help I needed. I could imagine the uncertainty my friends and family would feel about my decision now.

I shared my news with my friends and my parents and I cried some more. I cried because I did not know what to do, I cried out of self-pity and because I was angry and frustrated. I could feel anger inside, but I felt so overwhelmingly helpless. The stress was building in my head and despair was creeping into my body. I was so exhausted that all I could do was cry.

That Friday, the 26th of August, I wrote in my

journal, *dirty black Friday.* I experienced many of those absolutely desolate days. They always came on a Friday. I would cry uncontrollably. One of my friends, the same friend every time, would call to see how I was doing on these Fridays. She probably thought I was dying because I was always in the depths of despair when she called.

## NATUROPATH #3

I was still reading the book, *The Cure for all Cancers,* and I wanted to find a naturopath who did muscle testing. Muscle testing is a technique used by practitioners to find yes/no communication with the subconscious. I wanted to be checked for two things: parasites in my blood and high levels of metals in my body. My new yoga teacher knew of a naturopath who did muscle testing. I called his office and was able to see him that same day because of a cancellation. When that fell into place so easily it made me think I was on the right track. Once again, armed with my notebook and test results, I headed for another naturopath's office.

I found out that I did in fact have blood parasites and a high level of aluminum in my system. Not surprising, as I have always been somewhat of a sweaty person, especially the nervous kind of sweatiness. In order to keep the underarm perspiration levels to a minimum, I used an antiperspirant that was very high in aluminum. It had taken me years to find it and I had been so pleased for the last several years not to have sweaty armpits. I hadn't realized how these metals contaminated our bodies. *Had I taken my vanity too far?* Who decided it was bad to have sweaty armpits anyway? And what was I going to use to keep my armpits dry? One more thing my mind could not handle or worry about at this time. I used nothing for the time being. I showered every day; one would think that would be enough. The naturopath also informed me that I had a vitamin D deficiency. He told me breast cancer on the right side meant anger and resentment and on the left, not nurturing the self.

Mine was on the right, so once again I was hearing the same anger and resentment story. *How did they all know that? Why hadn't any of the doctors said anything about that?* The naturopath was thorough, but I wanted him to be more informative. I purchased the necessary supplements for the metals in my body and the blood parasites. I felt good knowing that my assumption was correct about the parasites and heavy metals but I also knew he wasn't quite what I was looking for as my healer.

**NATUROPATH #4**

Two days later, on August 31st, I had an appointment with another naturopath as well as an herbalist. I actually knew something now—I knew I was vitamin D deficient, had parasites in my blood, and high aluminum levels. I knew of a couple of different cancer treatment options and I didn't quite know which I would decide on.

Also, I was becoming more comfortable talking to different naturopaths and I could tell which ones I liked and which ones I didn't.

Once again with my blue notebook and test results in hand, I brought along *The Cure For All Cancers*. I wanted to see who knew of this book as it was helping me understand so much about this disease. I filled out a questionnaire, – about three pages of information relating to any health problems I had, the amount of alcoholic drinks I had in one day, whether I smoked, and so on. On the front page was the question: *What are you here for today?* I wrote on the line, "breast cancer." The doctor invited me into his office. As we walked down the hallway he read the questionnaire. We sat down and he looked at me and said, "breast cancer."

"That's what they told me," was my reply. I handed him my file of test results and asked him if he had read *The Cure For All Cancers*, which he had not. That was a little disappointing. He proceeded to scan my test results. Pen in hand, I was ready to begin my note-taking. When he looked up, I told him I had seen other naturopaths, none of whom could help me. I told him about the vitamin D deficiency, the parasites, and the heavy metals in my body. I told him I was looking for the "loop;" there had to be a loophole that I simply hadn't found yet. There had to be people who knew how to treat this with alternative and natural ways. He nodded gravely. "You have found the loop," he said.

I'll be the judge of that, I thought. "I want to be in charge of what I do and don't do," I told him. "I will decide who I see and what I do. I will be accepting other healing methods, as well."

He looked at me intently and nodded. "Wow! I think if I were in your situation I would handle it the same way you are. You are driving the bus here. I will guide you and help you in any way I can. You are in charge; don't let anyone tell you different!" I told him that I did not want to do chemotherapy or radiation or hormone therapy. He said that he understood what I was saying, but he also said, "We are not dogmatic!" I made a mental note to look that word up in my dictionary. He looked at me with his eyebrows raised. "Do you know what that means?"

"No," I answered truthfully. I didn't care if he thought I was stupid.

"It means we use all our resources. We may want to use everything that is available to us. Neither of us has all the answers but working together we will be able to deal with this situation. I would definitely suggest that you keep seeing the oncologist."

I was a little taken aback at this suggestion as I did not want to keep seeing the oncologist. I didn't like him. I didn't like going to the Cancer Agency and was not planning to use any of those other resources, even if they were available to me.

He told me about many different alternative treatments that were available. He also spoke of acupuncture and a man in the area who made a natural chemotherapy called Taxol; it was made from the bark of the West Coast Short-Needled Pacific Yew Tree. He also spoke of colonics and coffee enemas, as well as sauna treatments. I agreed to get some blood tests done (not covered by my medical insurance) and a saliva test so we could see what was going on with my hormones. Well over forty-five minutes later, I left the office feeling confident and relieved. I liked this guy; he really told it like it was. I had found the loop!

# Chapter 11

# THE HERBALIST

## Friend For Life

A couple of hours later, I was sitting in another office and speaking to an herbalist. Once again I went over my test results; the parasites, heavy metals, and vitamin D deficiency. She was interested, knew a lot about what I was up against with the medical system and I could tell she was knowledgeable about what my body needed. I was exhausted, stressed out, and running on adrenaline, but I had found another link in my chain of healers. As I sat and chatted with the herbalist, I felt as if I had known her all my life. She reminded me of someone but I couldn't figure out whom. She was a wealth of information. An hour and a half later, I was on my way with pages of information on burned-out adrenal glands and what to do to heal them, tinctures, and how to help the body heal. I felt stressed and exhausted but really grateful that I was finding my team.

The following week I had blood tests done for the naturopath. I also had an appointment coming up in the city with a medical doctor who worked in an integrated clinic. I wanted to be in touch with a medical doctor because I was on short-term disability from work and I needed a medical doctor to sign my forms. I had had my previous doctor sign my last batch of forms, but I knew I would not be seeing him again since I was not going through with the chemotherapy and radiation.

# Chapter 12

# JAKE

## Angel In Our Midst

A few months previous to my diagnosis one of our dogs, Jake, passed away. He was old and tired, and in his youth he had had a great passion for life. He loved to run and loved a good adventure and his true passion was swimming. Being a labrador retriever/ springer spaniel cross, he loved the water.

My husband and I often took our two dogs to the beach or to a lake. Jake was very intense and loved it when someone threw the ball into the water for him to retrieve. Having no children, our dogs became our children. It was very sad for us when he passed. Jake's birthday and mine were the same, so I felt we had a special connection. When we brought him home at eight weeks old, I held him on my lap in the car and he kept crawling over to my husband. They had a very close bond and love for one another. He was a beautiful dog with a beautiful spirit; he was very friendly and affectionate.

When Jake passed away, Molly, our other dog, and I walked through the forest together. I would think about Jake and get emotional because I missed him.

On our first walk in the forest after he died, we saw a big reddish brown moth, about two inches wide. It flew right in front of us and landed on a rock, and then it flew away. This was February, on the west coast of British Columbia, the middle of winter, so I thought it odd to see a moth at that time of year. It was the same colour as our Jake. As Molly and I walked through the forest, I imagined how I really wanted my life to be. I wanted to walk in the forest every day and feel happy.

When I had to work every day it was difficult to find the time to indulge in that hour's walk in the forest when I had to make dinner and keep the house. Besides that I was always so tired. The passing of our beloved Jake was a very emotional time for me, so I booked a week off work. Every single day Molly and I took an hour to walk through the forest. I came to absolutely love that forest. I felt so good afterward. Sometimes I felt as if I had figured things out in my life. Sometimes I wished and prayed and daydreamed that my place of employment would offer a voluntary resignation with a severance package for anyone wanting to move on. I imagined having a year off with pay and finding the perfect work that I loved.

At night I wanted to dream about Jake. I

usually did when someone died. Even when my parents' dog died, I dreamed of him running through the trees near their home. He was young again, and happy. It bothered me when I didn't dream about Jake.

I had heard about automatic writing and read about it. According to Richard Webster in *Spirit Guides and Angel Guardians*, automatic writing is a way of communicating with our guides using a pen and paper. The writing is directed by a power other than our conscious mind.

Now seemed like a good time to give it a try, so I got paper and a pen and sat very quietly, but all I saw on the paper was scribble. Then I could feel the emotion rise in my throat, missing Jake, and I put the pen in my left hand (not the hand I usually write with) and I asked if Jake was okay. The pen started to print words and it felt like something was guiding the words that were showing up on the paper.

It wrote:

*Jake is happy. Don't be sad, he is happy, he is swimming. He loves you, his mom and dad and Molly.*

Happy tears sprang to my eyes when I read it. That would be just like him to be swimming and having way too much fun to come and visit his mom in a dream. I felt relieved and satisfied that our Jake was in fact swimming and enjoying himself in heaven. It lightened my mood. I even felt impressed with myself, the way I got the message.

# Chapter 13

# INTEGRATED CLINIC IN THE CITY

## Unorthodox

Every once in a while I would doubt the way I was handling this thing called breast cancer and wonder if I was doing the right thing. Why was I so adamant about not doing chemotherapy, radiation, and hormone treatments? Why was it a given that so many women went forward and did what the doctors told them to do? Why was it different for me? Sometimes I didn't know anything anymore.

I heard about an integrated clinic in the city. It was on my list of things to look into. What a concept! Why didn't all doctors and naturopaths work together to help heal people? Actually, I knew the answer to that already. The drug companies' involvement by paying for all the studies reflects the notion that treating the symptom cures the body. There were few studies done about treating the body, mind, and spirit because there was no money in it for the companies.

I needed a medical doctor on my team of helpers to sign the forms from work; they would not accept a naturopath's signature. What a waste of money, to have to see a doctor just to get the forms signed, even though I was seeing a naturopath for my treatments. It didn't make much sense to me. I also wanted to see a medical doctor to relieve the little bit of doubt that nudged me now and again about natural treatments. *How could I know I was doing the right thing?* I decided to see what would happen if I tried automatic writing about the issue. So once again, pen in my left hand, I sat with paper and self-doubt, anxiety, and a little fear. Once again letters became words (which I could barely read at first) and a message was written on the page, suggesting I had the answer:

*We want to tell you to be careful about doing the chemotherapy. Don't wait for the judge. You be the one to say what goes here. We want you to see another way. We want you to see, sell the way.*

I knew I was grasping at straws, but I needed some sign or some way of knowing I was in fact listening to my own guidance. I honestly didn't know who to ask or how to alleviate the constant doubt that crept into my mind. If I asked someone what they thought I should do, I felt it was giving away my own power and responsibility. I just could not trust that anyone would know or believe, like I did, that I was listening to my body in order to heal myself.

It is easier when someone agrees with what we are doing. I didn't know who I could actually believe. Though it did seem to me that some of my friends believed in the path I was on for myself and my healing, I didn't tell anyone that I was doing automatic writing for a long time. I didn't really believe in it, myself. They would probably think I really was off my rocker.

I telephoned the Cancer Agency and postponed my chemotherapy class and chemotherapy start date. I told them I wasn't ready to begin yet. That was quite a process in itself. I had been told at the first meeting with the oncologist to recite the seven-digit number assigned to me whenever I called the agency; no need to give them my name. I *did* have a problem with that one! Imagine being nothing more than a number to them at the Cancer Agency. When I called I told them my name, and that *no, I did not have my number handy.* I guess they had to find my records the old-fashioned way, with my *name*!

I asked if they knew of an oncologist willing to work with a naturopath. The receptionist didn't seem to know or care and became defensive at the thought of someone seeing an oncologist and a naturopath. I was not aware that the combination was such an outlandish prospect; I thought it was a good idea.

With my notebook and test results in hand, I went into the integrated clinic to see the medical doctor. I found it interesting that they all meditated together, ate very healthy food, and the doctor was learning muscle testing. They had fireside chats some evenings, right there in the clinic, where anyone could come to listen and share. The doctor spoke of the body-mind-spirit connection (yes, really, a medical doctor). She thought we might explore my beliefs about work (i.e. why I hated it so much), the subconscious mind, and muscle testing. She told me about a book that focused on cells, *The Biology of Belief*, by Bruce Lipton. She talked about vitamins, and the possibility that my hormones were out of whack, though she used the term "unbalanced."

I asked her how doctors and naturopaths could work together in one building. Apparently the head naturopath had asked permission from the government and it had been granted. So there were five medical doctors working side by side with the na-turopaths. There was also a massage practitioner, a Reiki master, a holistic nutrition consultant, a sound and energy healer, and a traditional Chinese medicine acupuncturist. Wow, I was lucky enough to be seeing a doctor who believed in what I believed in! I could see her as many times as I wanted, but only for the healing of cancer. She could not be my regular general practitioner. After an hour and a half I finally stepped out of the building feeling very pleased and somehow lighter, in spite of the parking ticket I found on the windshield of my vehicle. It seemed I had indeed found my loop! I was relieved and happy. If she was the "judge" (from my automatic writing), I believe I had the 'okay' to keep following my path.

The next day I had an appointment with my naturopath for the results of the blood test he had ordered. I also joined a meditation class so I could learn how to meditate properly. I had always wanted to learn but never had the time or the energy to attend an evening class because I was always so tired. The following day I would be seeing my herbalist.

# Chapter 14

# SUPPORT GROUP
## #2

### Attitude

I decided to try the breast cancer support group one more time. This time I would try the other group, women who had had breast cancer in the past or were in the middle of treatment. There were about twelve of us and they spoke of tumour markers, blood tests, chemotherapy, and the side effects caused by certain medicines. It was a little overwhelming to listen as one woman told another about a drug she had taken. She called it by name and went on to describe all the details.

Once again, the leader of the group was very kind, she was plump with dark brown hair and pretty dark eyes, she had a gentle nature. The women all seemed to know each other quite well. Most of them were older than me. There I sat, again being the "new girl." I remembered being the new girl when we moved three times in one year when I was in Grade 3. It wasn't easy. All the other kids knew each other and I didn't feel like I fit in.

Now, at the support group, we took turns around the table as everyone either told their story or said, "Pass." When it was my turn I said I was doing natural and alternative treatments and that I believed there were other ways we could heal. One woman asked me what the statistics were on treating cancer using alternative methods and I told her that there weren't any statistics because all the studies were paid for by the drug companies and they only studied conventional treatments.

Another woman said her daughter-in-law had tried alternative treatment but it didn't work so she had to do the conventional treatments after all! I felt as if I was being bombarded with a huge wave of negative energy. Later, as I was driving home, I remember thinking, *If you call that a support group then maybe I'll just do this on my own. Why would I get together with them if they didn't support what I was doing?*

When I told my husband what was said at the support group and how I felt, he gave me an intense look. "Maybe you are not going for yourself—maybe you are going for them."

Maybe I *was* going for them, but I needed support for myself at this vulnerable time. I could possibly handle going only once in a while.

# Chapter 15

# NATURAL CHEMOTHERAPY – NO SIDE EFFECTS

## The Power and Healing Energy of a Tree

My naturopath had told me about someone who made a natural chemotherapy, called Taxol, from the bark of the West Coast Short-Needled Pacific Yew Tree. He had given me the man's telephone number. I researched the information on the Internet and then made arrangements to obtain some. When I met him he explained that it was made like a tea and he explained its origin. Apparently it has been widely used in other cultures for hundreds of years. Taxol, in its natural state, has no side effects and is a simple tea made from the bark of this tree. My dosage was one teaspoon every other day.

I realized one of the chemotherapy drugs the oncologist had suggested for me was called Taxol as well, also called Paclitaxel. I read the information about this chemotherapy drug that the oncologist had given me as it was on my list of chemotherapy treatments. The chemical is derived from the same tree, the West Coast Short-Needled Pacific Yew Tree. Other chemicals are added and then it is patented so that the drug company can make their money from it. Finally it is injected into a vein.

The information from the oncologist stated that Taxol (registered trademark) is partially produced from the bark of this tree. The side effects could include allergic reactions: Flushing, rash, itching, dizziness, swelling, or breathing problems, also mouth sores that could lead to bleeding gums which could lead to infection. Hair loss is common. All these side effects are from the other chemicals added to the original natural substance. It also contained alcohol so drowsiness might occur. Other drugs would be administered to help cope with some of these allergic reactions, one of which could also cause drowsiness.

I was tired all the time as it was. I felt like I was literally running on empty and had felt like that for years.

# Chapter 16

# MEDITATION CLASS

## Bathtub Full of Tears

My meditation class was very interesting to me as the teacher also discussed energy; how to feel our energy field and someone else's (without touching the other person) and how to protect ourselves from people who steal our energy and attack our auras on an energetic level. I had read many books on the subject, but to actually attend a class where everyone was comfortable talking about such phenomena was a thrill for me, to say the least. There were ten classes in all and I enjoyed each class immensely.

I didn't tell anyone that I had breast cancer and it was amazing how many of my fellow students picked up on the different energy in my armpit area, where they had removed the lymph nodes and a portion of my right breast. They could feel that the energy had been disrupted in those areas.

These classes were taught by the medical intuitive with whom I had had a couple of appointments. He was soft spoken, not a large man, with blue eyes. I had heard about him before this illness and was always very intrigued by this energy stuff and psychic learning. On one of my visits he told me that I didn't love myself. My question to him was "How do I learn to love myself?" He suggested a book to read which I put on my list: *You Can Heal Your Life*, by Louise Hay. He also told me to look in the mirror and tell myself that I loved myself. Okay, I could probably do that.

One late afternoon I was feeling very emotional and decided to have a bath. I was feeling chilled and wanted to warm up; a nice hot bath might do the trick. I felt very tired, worn out, and teary.

When I got into the tub I remembered what the medical intuitive had told me, that I didn't love myself, so out loud I said, "I love myself." As I spoke these words I burst into tears. Hearing these words echoing off the tub and water was shocking and I began repeating over and over that I loved myself. I found myself sobbing. Huge waves of sadness and loneliness washed over me as I kept repeating the words. Finally the sobbing ceased. I could feel a shift happening within. I knew in my heart, finally, that I did in fact love myself. I could believe it! It was as if my mind, body, and soul had connected; that *me, myself, and I* finally understood that we were all right here.

61

If we don't love ourselves then how can we love somebody else, and how can we accept anyone else's love for us? I felt connected and at peace in my being.

## Chapter 17

# BLOOD TEST RESULTS

## Forgive the Past

A couple of days later I went to the naturopath to get the results of the blood and hormone tests. Cortisol was below normal. Estradiol and progesterone were in the low range. Globulin was low. I already knew I had low thyroid function and had been on prescription medication for that for the past twenty years.

In my early twenties I had seen a doctor because I wasn't feeling well. I had been struggling with weight gain and felt depressed and lethargic. Usually an early riser, I was having a hard time getting out of bed in the morning and was always tired. He checked my heart rate, shone a light up my nose and in my ears and told me to say "ah" so he could look down my throat. Nope, nothing was wrong with me.

So I went to another doctor. I didn't like going

to doctors but I felt I had no choice. I didn't feel right. My energy was very low and I was starting to put on weight. This doctor said it was "maybe too much fork to the mouth." I was rather indignant about this because I had just come off a strict diet while training for a bodybuilding contest, so I knew how much and what to eat. I was still being careful about what I ate because it was normal to gain a few pounds after a bodybuilding competition diet. I was well aware of that. I was also still working out and running almost every day, so I was in good shape and knew something just didn't feel right with me. I had no energy, felt depressed, and just didn't feel good. I didn't know how else to describe it. I could also see that I was getting fat. I was insulted at his snide remark and I felt he was judging me; he didn't even know me.

The low energy and fatigue were debilitating. I went to another doctor who told me I was so brighteyed and bushy-tailed, he had no idea why I needed to see a doctor. I told him I felt depressed and was really tired and I had low energy, but I guess as long as I looked good, that's all that mattered.

I went to six doctors all told, before finally the sixth doctor had me take my basal body temperature for a month. The basal body temperature is the temperature taken the moment you wake up in the morning, before becoming fully awake, before moving, before anything. Mine was below 37°C or 98.6°F.

That was an indication that my thyroid was under active, and I began taking a thyroid prescription. The thyroid gland plays a huge role in the body; among other things it produces hormones that affect every organ and cell in the body, as well as heart rate, body weight, temperature, energy level and menstrual cycles. The thyroid is the centre of the lymphatic system, a major component of our immune system.

Over the years I had seen doctors for things like night sweats that had nothing to do with menopause; they had started off and on when I was in my early thirties. Still the doctors said nothing was wrong with me and that maybe I had too many blankets on the bed. These night sweats weren't from having too many blankets on the bed. My husband was always a lot warmer than me and he wasn't sweating at night. I was always cold and I still sweated through the night; I would soak my side of the bed and my pajamas. I guess nobody thought to check my thyroid and I didn't realize all the functions of the thyroid gland. We didn't have the Internet then. I remember reading everything available on the thyroid gland at the time and still not knowing a whole lot about it. Because the thyroid regulates the hormone function throughout our bodies, it made perfect sense to me that it not functioning properly may have had a lot to do with my not conceiving.

What I began to realize, though, is some of the doctors I had seen throughout my life were nothing more than stupid men that I had put my trust in. I had mistakenly thought they could somehow help me. I had gone to doctors and specialists for infertility problems. It is known that thyroid function is directly related to fertility, if conception isn't happening and a woman is taking thyroid medication one would think a *doctor* would have the sense to investigate that situation thoroughly. They all knew I was taking thyroid medication; every Doctor Tom, Dick, and Harry was willing to look up my private parts for clues as to why I was not able to conceive, yet not one of them took a look at my thyroid function in depth. I wish I had known more about this back then. Maybe I would have been able to have a baby. No wonder I didn't trust doctors or like them very much.

One day I remember saying "No more!" No more asking some doctor-man about my problem when all he would do would be to give me a physical examination—what in the world could he see anyway? An acquaintance told a story about a gynecologist who in social situations would talk about some of his patients in a very unprofessional manner, shall we say. He would talk about things he shouldn't have been sharing. Unfortunately for me, I had seen this doctor. It makes me feel disgusted to this day.

Maybe that was when I began to shut myself down, not knowing that I was shutting down my own immune system as well. Extreme cramps during my menstrual cycle was another reason I had seen doctors in the past. I took ibuprofen for three days, maximum dose, during every menstrual period for years because I could not tolerate the painful cramps. Night time was especially agonizing for some reason and because I needed my sleep so I could get up and go to work in the morning, I felt I had no choice but to take medication, even though I didn't like to take drugs for any reason. The pain was great enough to support my decision. I didn't know what else to do.

I had a blood test every year and my thyroid was supposedly within range. I had also seen a psychiatrist in my twenties for depression. I felt tired and really teary all the time. Once a week for a couple of months he sat and listened to me talk about goodness knows what, without saying a word. He thought antidepressants would fix me. I tried two or three different kinds, and each caused me to sleep twelve hours a night, and gave me constipation and grogginess that I couldn't shake. I never did feel any better. The day he gave me an envelope full of pills to help the other pills work better I went home and flushed them all down the toilet. That was the end of that psychiatrist and the antidepressants.

Now my naturopath had me take my basal body temperature every morning for a month to get my own reading on the thyroid function. Mine temperature was below 37 °C (98.6 °F) once again. I was still taking the prescription medication and the doctor had my thyroid tested by the lab every year, including earlier this same year. These were the highlights of the results: My adrenal function was almost non-existent, practically destroyed. That could have been related to my thyroid dragging along for who knows how many years. Adrenal function affects practically everything in the body, hormones includ-ed. My hormones had been out of balance for maybe for over twenty years. Maybe that's why I was not able to conceive.

No wonder I was so tired and depressed. My body had not been functioning anywhere near capacity for a long time. No wonder I got cancer!

# Chapter 18

# ONCOLOGIST VISIT #2

## The Wizard of Oz

On October 3rd I had to face that oncologist again. I didn't want to, but agreed with my naturopath that "we didn't want to be dogmatic." My husband came with me for moral support—I was a little afraid to go by myself. This time I was better prepared.

I still had that nervous, icky feeling and I really didn't want to be there, but I had a few questions up my sleeve. The nurse came in to weigh me and ask her dutiful questions. Once again, I did not want to answer her questions or get onto the scale. I knew my weight hadn't changed, even though I had no scale at home. I would have known if I had lost any weight. I wasn't going to do the treatments at the Cancer Agency anyway so there was really no need.

Of course I didn't tell her that. I didn't want

to sound too cheeky so I told her how much I weighed. Apparently she needed to see it for herself so I obliged. Yes! I thought, as I stepped off the scale. It was exactly what I said it would be.

When the oncologist came into the room I got an intense *ewww* feeling. My heart started pounding and adrenaline rushed through my body like a wave. He seemed defensive as he explained that standard chemotherapy reduces the risk of future reoccurrence. He told me that this is what studies done in the past have proven. Yes, he knew it was a synthetic chemical, but it improves the chance of cure. The goal is to live longer, he stressed. After three months post-surgery, the longer I waited, he stated, the more uncertainty, the less it would make a difference. The chemo travels to the cells and kills them. In 1977 it was proven that there was a larger survival rate for those who used chemotherapy.

When I brought up the subject of strengthening the immune system he merely shrugged. According to him, the immune system was not thought to have anything to do with cancer or the treatment of it because in kidney cancer chemo does not work. I sat there absolutely stunned at what I was hearing. My mind was reeling. I wouldn't have been surprised if my mouth were hanging open in disbelief. I remember looking at him and thinking, *W hat?* I wondered if he realized that nothing he was saying was making any sense.

He kept trying to convince us by explaining that when the immune system is totally suppressed for transplants, the patient does not get cancer. That was his reasoning! And therefore the immune system must play no role?! He did admit that they were experimenting with immune support for kidney cancer. I was at a loss about what he was trying to convey.

I could not believe it. Even as I write these words it sounds too far-fetched that he actually said those ridiculous things. But I took notes and I am repeating what I wrote that day in that room with that oncologist. I had had lots of practice taking notes by then! I wouldn't have been able to remember anything if I didn't.

I asked him what he believed in. His head jerked back slightly and he blinked once. "Data," he said. My eyes must have been the size of saucers at this odd reaction. Well, I might as well go for it, I thought. "But the data is only one-sided because the drug companies pay for the studies."

"Who told you that?" His tone was quite sharp. "No one told me." I wasn't going to back down. "I read about it, it's common knowledge." Oh my gosh! He didn't get it that there are some of us who actually realize where funding comes from for these studies. "Well, maybe you are not informed." His manner was quite cold, now. "After three months, time is almost up." He stared down at me. "There are two different kinds of people, ones that come in and do whatever the doctors say. Then the other kind, who

71

take complete responsibility for their choices, their treatment, and their cure." I asked my husband if he had any questions. "We are almost out of time, so please ask it," he snapped.

My eyebrows shot up. Oh, getting a little testy, are we? My husband asked what random studies mean and how they are done.

"Randomly controlled means they flip a coin as to whether it's natural or chemo." His tone was still short. "Random studies done with only chemo are still not totally accurate. The percentages of chemo studies that prove chemo works are based on random checking. They still haven't found a better drug to use. No studies have been done on the natural methods because there are no monetary gains."

He reminded me once again that we were running out of time. "Three months are almost up—are you going to go ahead with the radiation and the hormone treatment?" I was vague in my reply. My naturopath wanted me to keep seeing this person, so I pretended I still didn't know.

On our drive home I could not believe what I had just heard. Believe it or not, an ugly sliver of doubt popped into my mind. *Was I doing the right thing?*

I saw this oncologist three more times and I finally had the courage to go alone. I asked him if there was a blood test he could do because I had heard of others having blood tests for tumour markers and such. He looked at me like I was from outer space. "There is no test, he said coldly. " I was so confused— what were the blood tests everyone else was getting? I declined the chemotherapy offer, I declined the radiation offer, and then I declined the hormonetherapy-for-five-years offer.

# Chapter 19

# TREATMENTS

## Bathtub Full of Coffee?

My naturopath and I decided on intravenous Vitamin C drips twice a week. I also took vitamin C powder, 1000 grams and the teaspoon of natural Taxol every other day. Also, I was taking homeopathic and herbal supplements my herbalist had prescribed as well as a natural supplement for thyroid and adrenals. I also followed my naturopath's suggestions on how to support and heal the adrenals. I was to get enough sleep, do something pleasurable each day, move the body and breathe deeply, believe in the ability to recover, keep a journal, learn which foods made me feel bad and which ones make me feel good, eat lots of vegetables and chew food well, make whatever lifestyle changes I needed to in order to regain my health, take responsibility for my health, and take the supplements needed to heal.

I added meditation classes, yoga, and a class on energy healing to my schedule. I walked every day, ate very healthy foods like spinach, kale, and Swiss chard every week and I juiced my own vegetables; carrots, ginger, garlic, apples, beets, onion, celery. I also learned how important cracked flax seeds and flax seed oil are for us. I got lots of rest. I felt like I had a very full schedule.

At the suggestion of my naturopath, after talking it over with two girlfriends, and with great trepidation, I decided to have a coffee enema. Actually my girlfriends decided to do it, too. Of course, all of us would do it in the privacy of our own homes; we would simply know we had company doing this odd thing. We couldn't stop giggling and laughing about it at first, the absurdity of sticking a tube up our butts and filling the space with coffee. I had received the instructions from my herbalist and passed them around to my friends. One friend was familiar with the procedure and offered her assistance; my other friend and I declined her kind offer. I knew one thing for sure, I was definitely going to perform the task on my own!

Apparently enemas are an excellent method for detoxification. It works by stimulating the liver and colon, causing more bowel movements so the colon is not always full. The ancient Egyptians used this as preventive medicine. My friends and I had a few discussions about this before we took the plunge. I wanted to be clear about the instructions. My friend was in the same boat as me — neither of us knew what to expect or how this would all end up. She wanted to know if we should use organic coffee, or if regular was okay. Personally, I thought it was a waste of good organic coffee, but who was I to know? So we asked my herbalist. Sure enough we were advised to use the organic.

We were supposed to do this in the tub, naked of course. After gravity filled the colon with the coffee (the bag was hanging from the shower head), we were to massage the liver, which is under the right rib, then, after holding the coffee for as long as possible, we were to release it into the toilet.

My friend, who wasn't familiar with the procedure, is a person who needs to know *exactly* how to do something like this, even more so than I. Her bathroom didn't have a showerhead; it had a large tub and a separate shower, so she would be using her teenaged boys' bathroom. Her concern was that one of her two sons would come home early from work or school, knock on the bathroom door wondering why she was in their bathroom, and she would be discovered in the awkward position of trying to get to the toilet. We had to go over the directions multiple times. "OK," she finally said over the telephone, speaking very slowly and deliberately, pronouncing each syllable, "so, we are lying in the tub with our colons full of coffee and after massaging the liver we somehow climb out of the tub, while still holding the coffee within, get to the toilet and release the contents?" I could hear her concern over the telephone.

Well uh, yes, that was what I had understood also, as questionable as it sounded. Her other concern was what would happen if she couldn't make it to the toilet. To be honest, it was also my concern. I didn't know the answer, and I didn't even want to know the answer.

I visualized any cancer still hanging around in my body getting flushed out. The procedure was a success and we both managed to complete the task without any unpleasant mishaps.

I was in regular contact with my herbalist and also a healer who practiced specialized kinesiology; I wanted to clear my body of any blocked energy, which I believed had caused the disease in the first place. I had to visit the medical doctor at the integrated clinic to let her know how I was doing. I also spoke to a nutritionist and learned something from her: to eat smaller meals more often as it's easier for digestion. I already had a good diet. She also suggested making a pot of soup every week and eating it for lunch. I could take it with me in a thermos if I had appointments. That way I would have a healthy lunch whether I was at home or out and about. I began making a big pot of soup once a week and still do now. I must say I do make a good soup. Even my friends want to know how I make it, although they say it never tastes as good as mine. My mom would chide me; "*Toot, toot,*" (for tooting my own horn). But sometimes we have to say it like it is, even if it is saying something good about oneself. My mom makes good soup, too, so I come by it honestly.

I received five colonic treatments to rid my body of any "old issues." The young woman performing the colonics said she lost eleven pounds after her first colonic. I asked her why she chose this line of work. She said that for years she had had trouble eliminating and was grateful to find out about this procedure, which alleviated her situation. Because of her experience with 'not being able to go,' she knew she could be understanding and helpful.

Well, I didn't lose any weight, maybe because I didn't have the same problem she had.

I also had a couple of acupuncture treatments. As the naturopath stuck the needles into various parts of the left side of my body, he would say, "Do you feel that?" I didn't feel anything. "Do you feel that?" I continued to feel nothing as he inserted numerous needles into my left foot, knee, and arm. He looked at me in disbelief. Finally he started on the right foot, knee, and hand. I jerked and twitched involuntarily and felt an odd sensation. He said that was how I should have reacted on the left side, as well. That was energy flowing through the body. My left side was totally shut down. He told me that the left side was the Yin, or feminine side, and the right side was the Yang, or masculine side. Finally, we got both sides connected and running smoothly. Who knew how powerful those little needles could be? There must be some truth in that ancient method.

I was exhausted and tired, but wired, and I was going to do whatever it took to heal my body.

# Chapter 20

# KNOWLEDGE IS POWER

## Thank Goodness For Books

I have always been a bit of a reader, when I can find the time and I'm not too tired.

On vacations I would try to get into a good book. I like books about how our minds work and I indulge in self-help and inspirational books, in the fields of spirituality, psychology, psychic phenomena, health, and personal growth.

When I was sitting in the chair at the naturopath's clinic with the vitamin C dripping into my vein for an hour and a half, I chatted with some of the other patients. I was reading *Excuse Me, Your Life Is Waiting*, by Lynn Grabhorn. The topic was the why and how of the Law of Attraction. I found the book so inspiring that my enthusiasm spread to every person I came into contact with. I raved about "this amazing book I was reading" and insisted that everyone read it. Many people

I knew did read the book and I was amazed at how many of my friends just said, "Oh, yeah, it was good," but did nothing to change their negative attitudes. They just didn't seem to get it.

That book resonated with me and a couple of my friends. I reread it three times because I wanted to get all that good stuff in my mind and start living the life I have always dreamed of. I wanted my life to be different than it was and the book taught me how to achieve that, and also how to heal from this disease.

# Chapter 21

# MY JOB

## Who Made the Rules?

I had worked at my job for over twenty years, yet when I started, my goal was to work only five years. I was in my early twenties and delighted when I got this 'good job' that paid well. Back then, when I set out to get a job, I had been determined to get one that paid well. That was my top priority. I achieved that and was very proud of myself.

The job itself was a cashier position offering union wages, benefits, the whole nine yards.

It took a lot of practice to work well with the public. I could not believe there could be so many problems related to a person's groceries. It was also very shocking to me, how horrible and obnoxious people could be. There were very nice people, as well, and many of these kind people became my friends. It is also very odd how many apparently ornery, horrible people became my friends, too, after I learned how to deal with them and realized they all had really good hearts.

I got into trouble every so often when I began working with the public because I would say more than I should have. I was hauled up to the manager's office more than once for either not following the rules regarding the customers, or for standing up for myself.

It took me a few years to learn to just think of what I really wanted to say to someone who was being less than pleasant, while smiling and being gracious. Inside I was seething with anger at their audacity and rudeness. Standing at the checkout all day, dealing with one customer after another can really grate on a person's nerves after a while. Not to mention the back and shoulder pain and sore feet that result. Every job has things to deal with, I know.

Around this time I met and married my husband. We bought a small house and began renovating it. Well, my husband was renovating; I was constantly living in a mess since he never quite completed one thing before tearing apart another.

One year flowed into the next at my job and after five years I was offered an off-till duty, so I didn't have to be at the cash register every day, all day. I had a new job, displaying books and magazines, which I loved doing. It gave me purpose and something I could complete. I felt a sense of accomplishment, instead of facing that old lineup at the checkout that never ended. (I know, we make it look as if it's an easy job but trust me, it isn't.) I also began receiving extra weeks of vacation time as the years went by and I now considered myself a "lifer," along with so many others I had worked with for many years. What could I possibly do now to make the money I was making?

I had invested many years and now we had a mortgage to pay. This was my life. I knew my job well, and felt comfortable. I took a few weeks on stress leave over the years to help offset the difficult times, and before I knew it, twenty years had gone by. Some days were unbearable, though. *How am I ever going to get through this day?* I would ask myself this at the beginning of some days.

I simply could not stand it at times. Some days I imagined I would simply drop dead. I would be putting through someone's grocery order and then I would just fall over and die, or I would become a puddle of mush and goop on the floor. But it never happened. That day would finally end; I would drag myself home, still alive, only to face another day. I wished I didn't have to work there any more.

The years went by, times changed and the workload became more difficult. Management was cutting back on staff to offset the cost of running the store and there was less help. Customers complained in the lineups about how bad things were. Customers and fellow employees all seemed so unhappy it was unbearable. I felt the life force being sucked out of my soul. Then, out of the blue, I was diagnosed with breast cancer.

# Chapter 22

# WISHES & DREAMS

## The Best Me That I Can Be

Now on my walks through the forest I began to think about how I wanted my life to be and how I wanted to feel. I imagined how it would feel to work at something I really loved. I could not even imagine what line of work it would be. The thought of going back to an eight-hour day seemed unbearable to me.

I remembered, maybe ten years prior, vacuuming the house on my day off, wishing I didn't work where I worked, and a question came to my mind. If I could have any job I wanted in the world, what would it be? I continued vacuuming and thinking, *Hmmm, what would I really like to do?* At first I couldn't even imagine what I really wanted to do and then the answer popped into my mind. *I would like to be a motivational speaker.* But, I thought, I don't have anything to say nor do I feel motivated in my own life, never mind trying to motivate others. I could see myself on stage like Tony Robbins, getting people inspired about their lives.

I still didn't have anything to say and stage fright had taken its toll over the years, but I did need to work. I kept wondering what my work might be and how many hours a day I wanted to dedicate to it.

I decided that I wanted to find my *work*, as opposed to a job. I didn't want just any old job. I had already done that for a good many years. I wanted work that I loved, that I totally believed in, something that I was good at and could really immerse myself in. I practiced saying to myself, "I absolutely love my work!" I would say it out loud when I was in my house and when I was walking through the forest (as long as no one else was around) just to hear how happy my voice sounded, even though I was totally faking it.

I could imagine my work as some kind of one-toone communication. Not as a counselor or anything like that because I didn't have the schooling. Nor did I want to spend days, months, or years in a classroom trying to stuff my head with someone else's rules and regulations about why people think and do some of the things they do and how to make it all better. I didn't always believe what I heard or read and, having been through years of psychologists, psychiatrists, counselors, you name it, I knew they hadn't really helped me. I tried them all, attempting to stay out of the depression pit that always threatened. I did not know what work it would be but I held onto the faith that it would eventually present itself.

# Chapter 23

# SPECIALIZED KINESIOLOGY

## There Is Incredible Healing Power In The Human Touch

My herbalist recommended a specialized kine-siology practitioner she thought would be bene-ficial to me. Specialized kinesiology is the study of how our muscles, movement, and posture are affected by emotional, mental, and physical factors. It concentrates exclusively on restoring natural energy flow and movement through the body and releases any blockages with gentle body muscle re-education.

The practitioner was great and the work really resonated with me. I saw her six or seven times and found it very worthwhile. After the usual two-hour treatments, I felt really good. She worked with my energy and body and sometimes asked about events that had taken place at various ages in my life. It was all fascinating. One day she asked me if I had had a recent vaccination for something. I had had one about five years earlier, when it had been brought to my attention that I had missed a rheumatic fever vaccination as a child. "Well," she said, "your body didn't like it." I was impressed with the fact that she recognized this.

# Chapter 24

# MY BEAUTIFUL MOTHER-IN-LAW

## "I Just Want to Work" Rosa

My mother-in-law was also going through some tough times with cancer. She would have it cut out and then would be fine for a while. She was a very kind and gentle woman. She absolutely loved her family and was a wonderful cook. That year, I was able to spend several days with her, learning the basics of Italian cooking. It is a time I hold very dear to my heart as I felt very much part of her family and the feeling of belonging felt good. In the past, my job had taken up all my energy and there seemed to be no time to spend helping my mother-in-law or learning to cook with her.

Together with one of my sisters-in-law, I learned some special recipes that year during the Christmas season and we were able to understand how this woman created very yummy dishes for her large family to enjoy. I was grateful to have those days with her, even though we were both dealing with our illnesses. We didn't speak about our health issues, as her English was limited (but not nearly as much as my Italian). We managed to communicate very well through our love and respect for one another.

## Chapter 25

# TREATMENTS COMPLETED

## If He Walks Like a Neanderthal, Acts Like a Neanderthal, and Looks Like a Neanderthal, Guess What?

We got through Christmas 2005. I had a vitamin C intravenous treatment December 28th and was still feeling extremely exhausted and stressed out. I was still carrying quite a heavy schedule of appointments and getting vitamin C intravenous treatments once or twice a week. I also had some colonics along with the odd massage to move the energy through my body. I was seeing an energy healer, still going to yoga, dealing with the disability company (which was interesting since I wasn't doing standard treatments), and of course seeing the oncologist every month or so.

I was still tired and really low on energy. I wondered to myself when I would know I was finished with the vitamin C intravenous treatments. I had asked the naturopath some time before but hadn't received a hint of when he thought that might be. I was meeting up with a girlfriend one morning in January 2006 for some after-Christmas sales shopping and after dragging myself around the department store I complained to her about how tired I was and that I didn't want to go to the intravenous treatment that afternoon. "Don't go," she said.

I was somewhat annoyed at her words. *Don't go?* This was my life we were talking about here. I had to go! I had to do everything in my power to heal. I needed to know I was doing everything that could be done to the best of my ability to get through this. Don't go—humph, easy for her to say. She didn't have this burden to bear.

As I was driving home after shopping, her words came back to me and I questioned myself. *What if I didn't go?* I imagined myself getting my blanket and lying on the sofa with the television on, just resting. My whole body relaxed at the thought of this. I felt so good. Then I thought of driving to my appointment and I felt exhausted and teary. I called the naturopath's office and cancelled my appointment for that day. That was the end of my vitamin C treatments. I knew I was finished. Thank goodness my friend had spoken the words out loud about not going to my appointment. These words had come through her so I could question my self and it came to my attention to listen to what my body was saying. I am grateful my dear friend felt she could share the words I needed to hear that helped me move forward and listen to that small voice from within.

Later that same week I received copies of three letters sent to the surgeon and my previous doctor from the oncologist, stating that I had denied treatments of chemotherapy and that I had decided to not proceed with the hormone treatment option.

The letters stated that I had reported difficulties with low thyroid and low adrenal function in the past, that I wished to preserve my options with regards to fertility, and that at this point I was content to be discharged to my family physician for ongoing follow-up. Ideally, that would consist of breast surveillance with monthly self-examination, physician breast examinations at threeto six-month intervals and annual breast imaging. He was not sure who I was seeing for primary care at the moment as he understood that I was mostly seeing alternative practitioners. I was at substantial risk of future relapse of my breast cancer and any new symptoms should be regarded with suspicion; however, routine screening for metastatic disease would not be helpful. He had not given me a specific return appointment, but would be available to review me, should the need arise.

I was absolutely beside myself after reading the letters; the sheer terror that ripped through my body was astonishing. The fear drove me to tears as I wondered why they would send me copies of these letters, and why they thought I still might die. I cried and swore at that S.O.B. oncologist for once again creating such doubt, panic, and fear within me.

*Was I healed? How would I know?*

One of my dear friends and her husband joined my husband and me for dinner at our home that Saturday evening. As we sat after dinner, drinking our organic wine, I told them how I had come to decide that my treatments were finished -when my body relaxed at the thought of cancelling my appointment, but felt stress when I thought of going to the appointment. I was attempting to give them some sort of indication and reasoning about what I was doing and why I felt this way. I was feeling good about my decision and enjoying their company. All of a sudden my friend's husband started asking me questions. How did I know I was finished with my treatments? Did the naturopath tell me I was finished? How did I know the cancer was gone? He told me he had gone to see my naturopath and had asked all about me and how I was doing. To tell the truth I cannot remember everything he was saying to me. I had just finished saying how and why I had known I was finished— the audacity of him talking about me, my health and my situation to my naturopath! I saw red!

I am sure I was a little bit delirious with anger. I grabbed my letters from the other room, and I slammed them on the table in front of him. "You can damn well think like all the rest of them, if you like!" I probably said a few more choice words before running, sobbing, upstairs to my bedroom and there, instantly, I realized how much better I felt. I could breathe—the outburst seemed to have alleviated some of the stress that had built up in my body and I wondered what I was going to do upstairs in my bedroom while my guests sat at the dining room table looking at one another, wondering what in the world had just happened. It seemed I was becoming very aware of my true feelings and the need to express them was becoming more and more out of my control.

Eventually I went back downstairs. My friend gave me a hug and confided that they had been arguing recently about how her husband didn't listen. Her husband gave me a hug and said he only wanted what was best for me. We continued our evening as if nothing out of the ordinary had happened.

# Chapter 26

# COUNSELLOR #1

## Mona Lisa Smile

I figured I had better get my mind checked out again, since apparently anger and resentment were the cause of this thing they call breast cancer. After the dinner episode I figured it wouldn't hurt to get some insight into my reaction. Apparently it was possible for me to "break free from deeply embedded negative patterns." I was up for it. I really wanted to break free from whatever was making me so angry and frustrated all the time. I explained to the counselor that I had tried psychiatry, psychology, and hypnotherapy, as well as other counselors throughout my adult life, trying to shed my baggage, but apparently I still had it.

Here I was with breast cancer—obviously I still had some issues. The first question out of her mouth was, "What was your childhood like?" I couldn't believe I would have to tell my story one more time! That is what the other mind-fixing professionals had asked of me. I thought I was finally finished with the childhood stuff.

I filled her in on my perception of my childhood, including that I had dealt with it, accepted it, moved on from it, and that it was in the past. Now I was angry at having a quarter of my breast removed and I didn't think rehashing my childhood was going to solve the problem of my being angry most of the time and taking it out on my husband and others. Overeating was also an issue for me, especially at dinnertime.

I went through her program of six visits, felt great, and then thought, once again, I was cured.

I remembered seeing 11:11 on her electronics machine and, once again, wondered that number meant.

In March 2006 I was due back at work. I was still very tired and I could feel the anxiety building inside me as I readied myself for my first day back to work. I had been off work for nine months and felt there had been no time to rest. I had been on the go for the whole time and desperately wanted to rest. I felt absolutely depleted. At the suggestion of my medical doctor at the integrated clinic, I made an appointment with a psychiatrist to see if I could get more time off. The only problem was that the only psychiatrist I could see without waiting for months was at the Cancer Agency. That, in itself, gave me even more anxiety. I didn't want to go to the Cancer Agency, and what would the psychiatrist think of me, since I was not doing the conventional treatments?

I managed to get through a couple of half-days at work. I remember one time at the cash register, putting through a grocery order. All of a sudden I could not remember how to do a transaction. Before I left, nine months earlier, new computers had been installed at the checkouts and now my mind was going absolutely blank. I stood there and didn't have a clue what to do. I looked at the lineup, at all those people counting on me to get the customer through so they could pay for their groceries. It seemed the whole world was moving in slow motion, as if time were standing still. I felt like running away. As I stood there one of my fellow cashiers walked past my checkout. I asked her to help me and together we got through it. If it hadn't been for her, I might still be standing there, not knowing what to do. Or maybe I would have run away. I stayed away from the checkouts after that.

And then I found out that my workplace was offering a voluntary resignation package to all who were interested. I could hardly believe it. It was what I had been hoping and wishing for on my walks in the forest. I was so happy! I definitely would accept the offer, which would take effect in June.

The day of my appointment with the psychiatrist at the Cancer Agency finally arrived. I was so worried she would tell me I couldn't possibly be feeling this stress and anxiety because I didn't do chemotherapy. I thought maybe she wouldn't believe that I had a hard time coping with work because I hadn't gone through the Cancer Agency. I had heard them call feelings like this "chemo head" at the support group. They explained "chemo head" as a spacey feeling, like not being in the body, a tired-but-wired feeling, and forgetfulness, stress, and anxiety. I felt all those things, too, but I hadn't done chemo.

I used my Law of Attraction theory and imagined that, somehow, we would have a good connection, the psychiatrist and me, even though I had not gone through conventional treatment. I arrived at the Cancer Agency with my usual anxiety and sat in the waiting area until the psychiatrist finally led me to her office. I told her how tired I was and how stressed I felt. After telling her what had happened at the checkout, I explained that I was accepting a buy-out offer in eight weeks. I was so nervous, my mouth felt parched. Then she said, "You shouldn't be back at work yet! Everyone needs a year off after they have been through this!"

Even though I was sitting in a chair, I felt like I was falling through the floor. I felt weightless, as if I was floating in space. A huge weight instantly lifted off my shoulders. I was so grateful and so relieved, it brought me to tears. She went on to say she knew of a woman police officer who had just been through breast cancer and had needed a year off work. I was so grateful! She wrote a note for me to take into work that said I needed twelve more weeks off!

I drove home saying *thank you* out loud, over

and over, to the universe, to myself, and to my dog, Molly, who came with me every day. Wherever I went she patiently waited for me in the car. I was so grateful.

# Chapter 27

# THE PSYCHIC

## Seth's Message of Peace and Love

Later on, in that spring of 2006, I went to see a psychic. I had gone to different psychics over the years, maybe one a year or every other year. I was curious about my life and where I was headed.

This psychic had an interesting method of doing a reading—well, they all do—but this one was unique for me. She did automatic writing. I went to her home, we sat in her office, and she began to write large letters onto a page. She wrote page after page of what looked like large circular letters, then she stopped and read what was written and recorded it onto a cassette tape. It basically said that I had been some kind of prophet and teacher in previous lives and also in this lifetime. Women weren't allowed to learn so I had been persecuted for my beliefs and I still had some cell memory of that. I was to trust in my own inner guidance, that is where the truth lies. Healing of past life issues was the best path. My female troubles were caused by holding in anger and the frustrations of life. This creates *dis-ease* and must be released. I must teach others this lesson. The best is yet to be for myself. Many limitations travelled with me into this lifetime and it is imperative that I walk my chosen path and be in peace. In this life is good health and strength with myself and in my world. Others begin to follow and the teaching begins.

"How shall I release the anger and frustration from my body?" I asked her.

She wrote:

*The beginning is to see it, recognize it for what it is, where it came from, and what it has done to me. Next is to visualize it in a form (like a bubble) or cloud, enclose it, encircle it in a bag, box, or …? And visualize it being sent into the winds, the ocean, or into the ground or …? It must always dissipate into nothing so that it no longer exists as an entity. Then fill the space in my body and/or mind with love. Love for myself and positive energy in gold. Surround it in gold and it must always dissipate into nothing so it no longer exists. Fill the space back up with love.*

I asked what the numbers 1111 meant, that I kept seeing and noticing everywhere.

Answer:

*This is a time for her to be focusing on herself and walking her path to the spiritual self and her mission to teach and write about herself and her journeys. It is the reminder that "I AM;" that she has the message inside. She needs to focus and find it and to share. She*

102

needs to write of her personal journeys in book form. There was a class on psy-chic development, Susan needs to be aware of her gifts and talents, and they are many.

In the soon time she will take a class on psychic development. It will be of interest to open her to her higher self. The future includes the wisdom she keeps within.

My guides try to communicate with me but there is no answer, no response from me. They are always present, in the forest, trails, even in the closet. I need to open the mind for words and answers. Speak with no sound and their response is there. I need to focus not so much outward, but inward. Susan knows she is on her path and the time is now to make the investment of time and energy to learn and teach. In the soon time is the change in lifestyle that enables Susan to follow her passion.

I am to trust in self and move ahead with joy in my own growth and development, always looking within for answers and guidance. I have so much knowledge from past lives, healing, automatic writing, spiritual journey, teaching, people will see how I have walked my walk on the path through writing and physical and emotional healing and how I have overcome the issues in life.

I was instructed to start my book; writing all-inclusive past-life experiences will be an inspiration. Always know she is to believe in herself, trust in self and remain on her path.

To release the bubble is the next and most important step on my journey for without that there remains *the detour on my path. The bubble is to burst and the rainbow follows.* I was to trust in my self and go in peace and love.

Interesting, considering I didn't tell her I had an illness! At the end of the session, I told the psychic I knew how to do automatic writing. She was impressed—she told me to use it.

* * *

I began to feel the weight gain and lethargy of hypothyroidism again. I started to feel desperate because I didn't want to gain weight and feel depressed. My body felt heavy and sluggish, and my metabolism was not working properly. Obviously the natural thyroid and adrenal supports from my naturopath weren't working for me. I felt tired all the time and I could hardly stand it. The gnawing question haunted my days: *Was I really healed? How would I really know?*

After expressing my feelings about my thyroid to my herbalist, she recommended trying some herbal support. I tried it. I was beginning to feel desperate and I didn't want to go back to the prescription I had been on for over twenty years. Obviously it hadn't worked that well for me. I would try everything natural I could, hoping to find something to help me feel good.

My herbalist prescribed some homeopathoc drops. She explained that homeopathy is like an essence and works by nudging the body in the right direction, toward healing. The body takes over and re-members what its function is. It then knows what to do. The body responds by waking up what is in dis-tress, whether it's under or overactive.

I was willing to give the drops a try. She gave me the dose I was to take and, sure enough, I actually felt my thyroid kick in after some weeks of taking the drops. I felt good, the weight came off effortlessly, and the lethargy went away.

I wanted to see blood test results from the lab regarding my thyroid function and I needed a doctor to sign another form for work, so I telephoned a new doctor and made an appointment. This doctor, probably my age, was a woman. She reminded me a little of myself; there was something familiar about her. I liked her right away. Explaining carefully to her what I had been diagnosed with and the route I had taken to heal was like tiptoeing through a marsh. I had to tell her, without offending her and her profession, that I didn't want to do the conventional treatments. I had found a way to heal with vitamin C intravenous therapy and other natural means.

Her eyes welled up with tears, "I can't be your doctor if you aren't willing to do the conventional methods. My mother has just been through breast cancer herself."

"But I want you to be my doctor." Then I delicately explained that for the first time in my life I was meeting someone who I actually wanted to be my doctor and she was refusing me. I explained that the oncologist had said time was up after three months; close to eight months had already passed so I was pretty sure (and secretly glad) it would be too late to receive chemotherapy.

If I would just go and speak with an oncologist whom she knew, she would be willing to move forward with me as her patient. And because I genuinely did want her to be my doctor, I didn't disagree with the plan, but I certainly didn't make any promises. She would call me regarding the appointment.

I felt so much better about my thyroid; from there I went straight to the lab to get my blood taken for the test. Once again the doubt returned. *Had I done the right thing? Was I healed?*

A couple of weeks later, I was back at the doctor's office to get the thyroid test results. As I sat in the room waiting for the doctor, anxiety swirling in my solar plexus, I wondered if she was going to send me away when she recognized me. As she walked into the room my heart was pounding in my chest and adrenaline raced through my body.

"Sometimes we think we know when we don't," was all she said. She went on to tell me that it was in fact too late to see an oncologist and that she had read the latest finds concerning vitamin C intravenous therapy, which was considered a natural chemotherapy. As I sat in the chair I could feel relief washing over me, wave after wave. She told me to bring in any form I needed to get signed; she was there for me and my thyroid was fine. I felt as light as a feather, as if I could float on air. I had liked her from the beginning.

The kinesiology practitioner had told me about some natural adrenal support that my body absolutely loved (she found this out by muscle-testing me). When I started taking Ribes Nigram (now called Black Currant), two teaspoons a day, it tasted good. I took it for a few months and then one day it tasted really strong. It burned and tasted bitter as it went down. I was perplexed. I didn't like it anymore. I didn't really understand. I had noticed that I wasn't quite so tired anymore. I thought that maybe my body had enough of this adrenal support. I asked my herbalist about it. "Yes," she affirmed, "that is the body saying it doesn't need it any longer." I took it again later, then stopped, then took it again, then stopped for maybe another year. My adrenals are now healed, and I take it only periodically when I feel the need for adrenal support.

# Chapter 28

# INFRARED THERMOGRAPHY

## Rest In the Cradle

I had heard about infrared thermography, a new approach to breast screening providing digital infrared imaging to measure breast tissue function. It made total sense to me, as it doesn't compress the breast tissue and examines the whole chest, breasts, and armpit areas. I booked an appointment, knowing I wouldn't get results until six weeks later. My hopes were high and I was counting on the test results because I really wanted some proof so I could tell others that I was healed.

After waiting the six weeks, and then some, the test results arrived in the mail; my heart was pounding in anticipation. I couldn't decide whether I wanted to open the envelope or not. I wanted proof that I was healed but I didn't know what I would do if it showed anything other than that. With great apprehension, I took a deep breath and opened the manila envelope.

It advised that a qualified health professional was recommended to discuss the report and ongoing health care. *Analysis of the infrared images was impaired as the tylectomy had undoubtedly altered the regional vascular and nerve integrity, thus precluding any symmetrical comparison.*

It also stated that *there was an approximate 20 percent risk for confirming malignant disease at that time. The discernment of any atypical thermal features in a patient with a prior history of malignant disease should encourage additional objective evaluation and close clinical monitoring as there is risk for persistent malignant disease at the primary site and multi-focal malignance.* The wording was very technical and difficult for me to understand. Here is a summary:

*Atypical post-procedural thermology sign with equivocal risk for malignant disease in the cranial-medial quadrant of the right breast. Atypical benign-type thermology of the left breast. A comparative restudy is recommended in 90–120 days.*

So there it was in black and white. I still had cancer and I was probably going to die after all. I couldn't breathe. Fear gripped me by the throat and pulsed through my entire body. It pounded in my head. *This was it—I had lost.* My mind was racing— *why had all this happened only for me to die?* A friend of mine, at my suggestion, had also done a digital infrared imaging, as had one of my sisters-in-law. Shortly after I reviewed my results, my sister-in-law telephoned to ask if they had arrived yet. I told her they had not; I could not quite deal with telling anyone what I knew.

When I finally told my husband, later that day, he said that I could still do chemotherapy. I screamed at him that I would rather die; I was not going to go through this again! He still didn't really know me after all these years.

The next day I walked with a friend along the beach and I told her about the results. She didn't miss a beat. "When were those tests done?" she asked. They had been done two months earlier. "You don't still have cancer; a lot has happened since then. You don't have it anymore." I cried for the whole hour we walked. I was so exhausted; my mind simply could not take any more stress. I knew I was not going to go through all this again, in any way, shape, or form.

Later, I did an automatic writing. It revealed this message:

*Release and visualize what you want. Release, release, stop holding it within, the detour will persist until you release, your choice.*

I asked: How will I know I have released?

The answer: *You will know by the way you feel. You will feel free all the time; no time will you not feel free. Yes, you know what is left, it will be OK. It will be good, not to worry.*

*It is when you aren't truthful; secrets are the cause of cancer. Let them out, let them go, who needs them? Be in truth always, never give that up. Get them out, release them, it harbours dis-ease. Do not be afraid.*

*You need not worry about your body, you need to release, and you need to tell, no more secrets now. Help everyone to release. You know how, you will. Today is when to begin, now. Share what is stuck inside you, tell, tell. You must do this to know how to release. Do it, you can, you must.*

*We want to tell you to free your soul. The unfolding will soon begin. Patience is called for, all will be well.*

I asked what love was:

*Love is when you find in yourself the reason to be. You cannot have your total self without having the experience of love, that is why finding it and looking for it is also your life mission. Always know we mirror each other. Really look at the other and you will see love mirrored back. If you don't look then you miss it and that is what it is all about ... love.*

*Look within, your answers are there. Listen to yourself, listen to your heart. Never look back, only forward and beyond. Never give up a chance to love.*

*We want to tell you to be cautious of your thoughts, only what you want, not what you don't want. Free your mind of any negative thinking, practice. Share what we tell you. Only think of what you want, monitor your thoughts. We want to tell you to practice, keep thinking and monitoring your thoughts.*

*We want to tell you to be more of yourself today, stay with who you are. Let us guide you, hear our message. Consider another view; take a close look at what it is you truly want. Be conscious, listen to yourself, peace, contentment, happiness, love, joy, everything, you can have it all. Be you. Believing you can*

111

*have all you dream of is the difficulty. Believe. Believe in happiness; believe in a wonderful, fulfilling life and you shall have it. Feel your wisdom from within, keep releasing and let yourself feel the love in your body, you are on the path. Heal your body, heal your soul and heal your spirit. You will live in peace and joy. Live your life well; leave behind what you must, and live, live.*

*We want to tell you to heal your body by opening your soul to another. When the love is mirrored back you will release the negative energy you have locked in. The healing begins and the future begins to unfold, go in peace and love. Love is always the answer, for all people, tell what you know.*

*They must always ask for what they wish. They must ask with clear understanding. Love is always the answer. Be in love and peace.*

My anxiety began to retreat as this wisdom and understanding revealed itself to me; I told my friend what my automatic writing had said about secrets, so I told her all my secrets and I cried. I knew in my heart she didn't judge me and I was so grateful. She also told me all her secrets and I felt no judgment, only compassion.

I made an appointment with my original naturopath who was recently back from maternity leave. I wanted her professional opinion about the results of the infrared imaging and knew she would be able to read the report and explain what I wasn't able to understand. She indicated that it was only the first thermography report and they always need a second for comparison.

Also, that indication of cancer could possibly be from the surgery itself, because it takes time to heal inside. It could take up to five years. Possibly the scar tissue needed to be broken up by massage with castor oil.

I knew in my heart that I was healed but I took another thermography test six months later. The results revealed: *A moderate decrease in the extent and calibre of the described atypical vascular-like pattern and the analysis of the infrared images is impaired as the tylectomy has undoubtedly altered the regional vascular and nerve integrity, thus precluding any symmetrical comparison.*

In other words, because of all the nerve damage from the surgery they would need ongoing compar-isons. Because I knew in my heart I was healed, I haven't felt a need for any more imaging.

# Chapter 29

# PERSPECTIVE

## Follow My Truth and Let Others Follow Theirs

One morning in June 2006, I awoke with the memory of a dream about perspective. I remember waking up with the words, "You have better perspective now." I had no memory of the dream itself, just those words. I remember thinking, *W hat an odd dream.* I had never had a dream like that before. I didn't know what I was supposed to have a better perspective of; I didn't really understand any of it.

Three nights later I had another dream. I was cleaning a car windshield in the dream and my friend was looking at me through the windshield. "This is a sign," she said. OK, I thought, once again not knowing what the sign was. When I woke up, I remembered the words, "After the year is up … happiness, peace, joy, freedom." I wrote it all in my journal. But I didn't understand it at the time.

Later, when I thought about those odd dreams, I got the whole picture. I could see myself in the vehicle, looking out through the windshield at my friend, and then I could see my friend in the vehicle and I was on the outside looking in at my friend. It was showing me how my perspective changed depending on where I stood (or sat) at the time. Interesting, but I still didn't understand why I had been shown that.

\* \* \*

I met a woman around that time who had breast cancer. She wasn't doing very well.

Since she lived near me and also had refused conventional treatments, the doctor at the integrated clinic asked me if I would connect with her. I was delighted to speak with her. I had very much wanted to connect with someone else who thought the way I did and who was choosing an alternative path. I looked forward to the phone call. We chatted for over an hour; we felt like we had already known each other. It became apparent after long conversations with her that she had not wanted to pursue conventional treatments and that she had chosen (in my opinion) to allow fate to decide her outcome. She was bedridden, couldn't use her right arm anymore, and was on pain management. Her right arm was in a sling and double the size of her other arm. On her own spiritual path, she had written a book and had made a CD of her beautiful songs.

115

We had many conversations. She was the only person I could talk to about the automatic writing, my guides, angels, energy, and the other metaphysical phenomena that I was experiencing, because she believed in the same. We seemed to understand each other and knew on a deep level that our connection was for a purpose: We were to help each other through this part of our lives. I asked her if she wanted an automatic writing. She did. Here is what it said:

*She needs to take care of her small child within her. Tell her to stop treating herself badly. Change how she thinks and views things. See and feel what is real. Do not let any one tell her less. She needs to release much anger. She can release it. She must or live again and again with it. Now is the time. Let her be taught. Let her listen. She must act now. She must release.*

She never released it. We didn't know how to release the anger and we didn't know how important it was. I didn't know how to help her live. She told me later that she was estranged from her family.

One day I told her it seemed I was waiting and waiting for my life to begin. She said she had just read something about waiting, *that there was no time for waiting, a new life awaits, a rebirth of our spiritual lives.*

So I waited for my new life and the rebirth of my spiritual life. I waited, and waited some more.

We became very dear friends in the short time we knew each other. Our connection was beautiful and it helped me to understand the importance of letting go and forgiving. She passed away six months after we met. I understand it was her choice. She chose her exit. I am eternally grateful to have known her; I still hear her little giggle.

# Chapter 30

# FEELING LOST

## Amazing Grace

On my walks in the forest I asked my guides, the angels, and the universe for happiness. I asked for joy even though I didn't know what joy was or how it would feel. I also wanted to find work I loved. I prayed intensely that I would release whatever I needed to release. I thought I obviously needed to release something because I had what they call breast cancer. It had to be some kind of indication that something needed my attention. I also thanked the universe every day for my healing.

I loved walking in the forest with Molly. Sometimes she would take a long time sniffing at something interesting and I would feel annoyed at having to wait for her. She was off-leash but was always good and stayed close by. She was somewhat shy and didn't want anything to do with other dogs or people. She only loved *her* people. I had rescued her when she was a year old; she had been my little dog ever since. With emotional problems that in some ways mirror my own, she tended to get a little bitchy once in a while; she was very decisive about who she did and didn't like.

As I waited for her to finish sniffing one day, instead of feeling annoyed, I began to look around at the trees, really looking at them. I looked way up toward the sky to see if I could see the treetops. I looked closely at the magnificent trunks of the Douglas firs and the branches that stretched outward, reaching as far as they could. Giant protectors of the forest, their branches extended like angels' wings. They were all so magnificent, just standing there, day in and day out, for years and years. It was all amazing when I really thought about it, and I stood in wonderment at how beautiful everything in the forest was. All the different colours of green and brown blended perfectly together. If my dog hadn't stopped to sniff so intently, I might have missed the beauty of that magnificent forest.

On windy days some of the trees creaked and groaned. It sounded as if they were singing. They reminded me of the whales. It was all very awe-inspiring. Almost daily I thought about my dreams and wishes of healing and releasing the negative energy in my body. I would receive guidance, or ideas, or some kind of inspiring message.

It was a constant struggle to stay out of the great depression pit that always lurked nearby.

Throughout my teenage years and all my adult life I had struggled with it. I had gone to psychiatrists, psychologists, hypnotherapists, counselors; to try everything I could to not let myself get completely lost in depression. I tried hard to be happy. I didn't know where happiness was or how to get it, but I desperately wanted it.

I was miserable. I hated my life, my job, and I even hated myself sometimes. Loneliness was a constant companion—not that I didn't have friends, I always had friends, and loved my friends, but a deep sadness and loneliness dwelled within me and I could never shake it.

The emptiness inside me was so all-encompassing that it threatened to swallow me up. It pulled at my being like a strong undercurrent in deep, dark waters. If I kept my mind busy I could keep it at bay. When I was in my teens I read books, wrote poetry, rode my horse, and was in a 4-H Beef Club. I had a good life, or so it seemed, but happiness always eluded me. How I longed to be happy. But it was never within my reach.

As I grew up, my parents mentioned a few times that "You cried until you were two years old." Maybe I never had been happy. I was also a very sensitive child, overly sensitive, one might say. When I was five or six years old my parents would ask, "What is she crying about now?" When I was a teenager I could not watch a sad movie or see an injured animal, and if someone died, well, forget about it, I cried. I knew I was oversensitive; I couldn't help it; the tears seemed to lie just under the surface all the time.

Finally, by the time I was in my thirties, I could sometimes get a handle on it. I learned how not to cry. If I breathed deeply and quickly thought about something else, I could hold back the tears until the feeling passed. I was so proud of myself; finally, I had control of my emotions.

Finding the job I wanted after graduating from high school and marrying a kind man, albeit a man who kept his feelings and thoughts to himself, but a man who adored me, gave me a sense of security. We didn't exactly have a very communicative relationship but I knew he loved me. Who wouldn't be happy with all that? I thought having my own home would make me happy. I loved my home, but happiness still wasn't within me.

\* \* \*

As spring of 2006 began to warm up, Molly and I walked to the beach so she could go for a swim. Our other dog, Jake, who had passed away, had taught her to swim and love the water years before.

I felt so inspired when I walked on the beach or through the forest; answers would come right to me. I would ask the angels to take all the negative thoughts and feelings out of my body, just as the psychic had described in the writing. I asked myself to release whatever I needed to release and thanked them for my healing. I gained insight on problems from the past and sometimes even on a friend's issues. I began to imagine my work and how I wanted my life to be. I imagined myself doing one-to-one work, possibly in a healing centre, not touching, just talking. I had no idea what sort of work it might be but I knew that whatever it was, I would love it. It would be my *work*, not just a job.

I started doing automatic writings for insight every day after my beautiful walks in the forest.

*We want to tell you that patience is called for; the unfolding of events will begin. All in due time, must not rush the process. We are looking out for you, you are safe, we need you to be patient, think of what you want. It will be, allow it all to unfold, hold on to the love.*

*Hold on to the strength within at this time. After the sadness is joy, keep the faith; you know it is right, your journey must continue as planned. Let the process begin to unfold, it will be good, great things are coming to you. Be in the now, you will be joyous, you have freed many in this process. Afterwards you will see how wonderful this is for all. Rejoice in your courage.*

*Good, happy times are on the way; your life work shall begin on many levels. Joy and gratitude are yours.*

*The sadness going through your body is a form of release. Do not wish it away but feel it, look at it, where does it come from? It is only you and your thoughts and feelings of how you are living your life. Take a step up back to your dreams. They are still with you. Let yourself feel your dreams; it is OK to let the sadness out. Soon the sadness will dissipate as you begin to really live your life to the fullest.*

*You are safe. We hear your tears, soon your eyes will dry and you will feel the joy once again. Let the tears fall a while longer. We are here for you; release the sadness all will be well soon. Remember the happiness is not too far away. It awaits you; move through this pain on the other side is gladness. Loneliness need not be a self-created fulfilled prophecy.*

It was a relief to know my guides knew of my sadness and they had a handle on it so to speak, because I sure didn't.

# Chapter 31

# RESENTMENT

*"Just because it's bad news for some people doesn't mean it's bad news for everybody."*
Bob Ryde

I felt good when I was walking through the forest or at the beach, but when I arrived at home I felt utter emptiness and a deep loneliness. I had no idea what to do with this feeling and didn't know how to describe it to my close friends. I called it the *ewww* feeling or the icky feeling. It was a feeling so deeply sad and desolate; my solar plexus felt raw, exposed, and vulnerable all at the same time. It felt like a gaping wound that was so tender it needed constant guarding and protection. Some days I looked around at our house, still in disarray from my husband's constant renovations, and felt total despair.

Before finishing what he was working on he would start tearing apart another room (we are talking about moving walls here). My husband is a master of that kind of work. He works on our home and also works his full-time job. To some, he is a husband to be envious of — apparently, not all husbands know how to do things around the house. "It will eventually all be brand new," I've heard more than once. I should be glad he knows how to do these things. Unfortunately, I am a person who wants everything to look nice. I like clean and am fine with things the way they are, or with minor changes, at most. I like to paint and decorate and have it all look good. It is very difficult to decorate and have things look good when the walls are two-by-fours and there is no drywall yet, never mind a wall to paint.

I was exhausted from looking at the mess day in and day out. Everything looked ugly and we would disagree about what should be torn apart and moved, among other things. With moving walls, ripping up floors to lay hardwood and granite tile, comes expense. Here I was on short-term disability, seeing healers not covered by any medical plan, my husband kept spending money on more renovations, and still the house was a mess! He was doing what he thought was best but it was making me uneasy. We never had a good, communicative relationship. Talking about money brought anger out in both of us, as our opinions differed.

I began to feel more and more resentful. I was finally not working and not running around trying to heal myself. I could actually rest, be home, and figure out what I wanted to do for work. The house was ugly and half-finished. I hated it. I was to the point where I just wanted him to complete what he had started, but he disregarded my suggestions. More walls were taken apart, only to be rebuilt inches from where they had stood. I was beside myself; I wanted out of this marriage where I didn't have a say in anything!

I could feel the frustration building inside me once more. I felt I had no say, no control, as if I was invisible. He was indifferent to anything I wanted and it was going to be only his way. We argued all the time. I told him I wanted a divorce and wanted to sell the house, but in reality, how could we sell it when it was torn apart? I felt trapped, alone, and useless. I felt as though I was tied to a very long tether that bound my hands. I could do whatever I wanted -as long as the tether reached that far. The price of security for me was freedom. When we take responsibility for our own lives no one can challenge our security. The wisdom began to flow through my automatic writing, the writing in my journal, and on my walks.

Through the employment office I heard about a two-week course that involved aptitude and personality tests to find out what motivated us and why different personalities preferred one kind of job over another. The test results were expressed by colour categories.

After two weeks in the summer of 2006, it seemed I didn't have too much to offer in the way of skills. Wow, one would think working with the public for over twenty years would earn a few credits along the way, but no. The teacher agreed. I could be a waitress or a cashier, and I desired to do neither. So now what? At least I had a personality, even though it didn't completely fall under one colour category. I was pretty much a mix of all the personality colours.

I bet that if we mixed them all together they would become the colour of mud. Or on the other hand, if I lined up all my personality colours in a row, I could almost imagine them creating a rainbow. Once again it seemed I just didn't fit in anywhere. There were all these categories— personality, interests, and such— and everyone else fit somewhere except me.

I began to write this book, even though I had no idea how to write a book.

\* \* \*

Since he didn't hear me, talking to my husband had been a challenge. Usually if I said something he simply didn't reply. He ignored me and I hated being ignored. It really got on my nerves, especially when later he'd say I hadn't told him.

I tried to have a conversation with him one day and I asked if he was happy. "No," he said. I tried talking with him more but he just got angry. I told him I wanted to live alone. He said nothing, the angry look stayed on his face. I felt lonely all the time. My husband and I argued constantly; it seemed the only time he would speak to me was when we argued. I felt such sadness and longing for more meaning to my life. It angered me, and suddenly I could understand why someone would end her own life. Sometimes the pain seemed unbearable. Here I had my chance to leave this planet, having breast cancer, and I had done everything in my power to stay ... and now, I wondered why.

Many days I went to the negative, doubtful, empty, depressed, lonely, self-pitying, dark place in my mind. I wondered about everything from choosing the right cell phone plan to how I would know if I were really healed. I felt that *ewww* feeling; I was full of fear, anxiety, and doubt. I prayed every day, *Please help me release this negative energy.* Some days I just said, "Help me, help me, help me," hoping the angels could hear my prayer. I felt unmotivated, lonely, sad, depressed, and I was unable to sleep at night. I felt as if I was waiting for something, but not knowing what, always waiting. My life was a great big empty nothingness.

My automatic writings during this time said:

*This is all for good, you will see, all your dreams and wishes will be. Be patient, just Be, we want to tell you that you will be so free and happy soon. Persevere; it will be so worth it! Do not rush, all will come to you in due time. Go within, shine your light; find your place of peace.*

*You must share what you know with all you know. You shall have great success spiritually as well as materially. You have grown your knowledge, your self is strong, you have the courage to live your life in an amazing state. You must practice what you know. You are free; you shall have all you desire. Keep the dream, keep the faith.*

*Be still, go within and look at what you need to do to let your life move along. Your purpose is to know when something does not feel right. You need to live your life in joy and gladness. You need to grow to find it.*

Through all the emptiness I was experiencing, I listened to what my guides and angels were telling me and trusted their guidance.

# Chapter 32

# VULNERABLE

## Mind Discipline

Often I wrote things down that came into my mind. On one occasion I wrote about all the things that made me feel vulnerable. I remember doing an automatic writing afterward and the writing told me:

*We want to tell you to decide what you are willing to feel vulnerable about in your life. You have the choice to feel vulnerable or feel empowered by your body and your mind. Try to choose empowerment for a while and see how that works for you. You have the choice. Empowerment will move you ahead in your life.*

I added this afterward:

*Empowerment will also keep us living. As we create and find our own empowerment that good energy and good vibes are sent out to the universe to help bring us our dreams and wishes. We need to find where our empowerment comes from. It must come from within; no one else can give it to us. We cannot get it from anyone else. Our empowerment is our own.*

How could I have been writing that in my journal while I still had a life of such disempowerment and depression?

Automatic writing:

*We want to tell you that you will have all your wishes and desires. Patience is still needed. All is very well; you have much love in your heart. You learn your lessons well. The pain in your stomach will subside, better to feel the pain now, sooner than later. You will be glad later, keep your dreams, they are so near.*

*Find peace in your mind. Develop the need for tranquil times of continuous soft feeling for yourself and others. Rest. Rest your mind at this time.*

I asked about 1111 and the response was:

*This is a code to remind you to do as YOU think. Keep your mind free, not negative, do anything you need to keep the positive, the Light.*

These sad days seemed to bring out some kind of wisdom in my writing:

Maybe we need to make changes in our lives when we get cancer. We need to really be clear with ourselves, about what is causing our dis-ease.

Somebody told me about someone else who had cancer and had undergone chemotherapy and radiation. Three years later the cancer was back. I wondered if she had changed anything in her life. Sometimes we don't even realize we are not happy because either someone has told us that we should be happy, to look at all we have, or we have told that to ourselves. But possessions are only a bunch of stuff. They do not bring fulfillment, joy, happiness, or life. When we get cancer, we need to get real, speak the truth, and be honest with ourselves. We need each other as well. Our dear friends help us to see ourselves; they are all mirrors to our soul. We need them and they need us. Together we can heal ourselves and each other. Alone we cannot, because we cannot see ourselves. Like a mirror, a friend bounces our reflection back to us, allowing us to see ourselves from a different perspective. Otherwise we only see ourselves and our lives from our mind's point of view.

A friend went to see my herbalist for some of her own issues and borrowed *The Secret*, a movie about the Law of Attraction. We immediately sat down and watched it together. It goes into great detail about how and why our lives are the way they are and what we can do to have all we desire. It explains that what we think about is what we create in our lives. I was riveted to my seat as I watched it. I wanted to hear every word they were saying. I needed to change the way I thought and the things I thought about, just as was suggested in the book *Excuse Me, Your Life Is Waiting* by Lynn Grabhorn. I had read that book three times during my treatments.

Finally, here was an answer to my desolate life – if I could just get my mind to shift, to believe I was in fact healed and happy. In the meantime, here was something I could do to change how I felt. I would practice. I watched that DVD every single day for more than thirty days. It always made my mood lighter; it gave me something I could hold on to as I tried to change my life. I watched it so many times I could practically recite it word for word, and still, some days the dread and loneliness crept up on me and I felt the agonizing raw pain in my being. I just couldn't shake it.

There was no happiness in my life, no fun, and nothing to laugh about; it was so sad and dreary.

I tried to make a list of all the things I loved. At first I could not think of anything. I simply could not remember. Finally, three things came to me: my bed, my dog, and my glass of wine with supper.

Day after day I sat at home with my mind racing. There were so many things I could do around the house but for some reason I couldn't get motivated. I went for walks, either on the beach or in the forest, and insights about my life often came to me. One day on my walk I asked the universe why I felt such anger toward my husband. The words that came to me during my walk were, "You have no voice." Instantly I remembered how often I had said to him, "You just don't hear me." I felt that he never allowed anything I said to matter. He didn't hear me, therefore I had no voice. The psychics I had been to in the past had told me I don't speak up but I had never understood what they meant. I thought I spoke up. I really didn't know what else I could do to be heard.

I felt stuck in life. Some days I just sat and did nothing. Nothing felt right, everything felt wrong. Some days I sat and cried. I constantly had the *ewww* feeling. I wondered if I did, in fact, still have cancer. I hated the way I felt, I hated everything.

Automatic writing:

*We want to tell you to not be impatient; you have done so well, soon your life will have meaning and purpose once again. Be in this moment and learn this lesson, you need to be in this moment for your life to begin. Being is the key.*

*Be true to your beliefs and pass on what you know.*

*Your sharing helps the learning of others, keep telling what you know. Soon it will show up in your life, so the people that have walked this part with you will see. You need to do as we ask. Next steps share what you know about wishing and dreams and desires. Use your passion for your self, find it within and dream your best dreams. You will succeed; you have so much knowledge, share it.*

*Be true to your feelings. Feel what you feel, don't shut down, your self needs to feel what you feel, this shall pass. Rest your mind today, tomorrow will be better. Honour your feelings, patience is called for. You are in need of happy times, ask for them, you need to find joy and inner peace, you will.*

*You are on your path to success, monetary fulfillment, and success in your health and love for people. You are to share what you know with others along your way.*

*You know truth; you must teach others what you*

*know. Just Be. Keep your mind in the now. Allow. This will allow you to receive. Find your joy, it is within, you already possess it. You are joy.*

My guides encourage to do as they ask, to be in this moment, even though it was not comfortable to feel what I was feeling in this moment. They still wanted me to dream and share what I was learning.

# Chapter 33

# SEXY DISEASE

## Pick Myself Up,
## Dust Myself Off

I went with a friend to the local bookstore one day to hear a talk about reorganizing. My friend is an awesome organizer and she was looking to possibly make a business out of helping others organize their homes.

The bookstore is where I heard about redesign — using the furniture and accessories a home already has to decorate and enhance its comfort and beauty—so I took a course in redesign and staging a home for sale. I had always loved using what we had to make a room feel comfortable. Of course, in my case, it would have been nice to have a floor and real walls to play with instead of plywood on the floor and no walls. But decorating was at least something I was interested in and it kept my mind off the feeling of nothingness that loomed over me like a great dark shadow. I thought this might be my new 'work' that I was searching for. It was something I loved to do and had been doing it for a long time in my own way.

The first time I heard breast cancer described as the "sexy disease," was during a conference I was attending with a group of women. My mouth dropped open—*had I heard her correctly?* I thought I was going to lose my mind when I heard those words coming out of a woman's mouth. *How could having a part of the breast cut off be sexy?* I began to shake. I swallowed back the lump that instantly arrived in my throat and I took several deep breaths. I asked a woman sitting next to me what the other woman had said, as I could not believe what I had just heard. When she repeated the words, I had to leave the room. I found a stairway where I could cry and allow my body to relieve some of the anger and frustration that once again began to build up.

Obviously that woman had not had the privilege of experiencing this thing they call breast cancer. I had been pushed beyond my capacity and could tolerate no more. I stood there in that stairwell and after I stopped sobbing, I wondered what it all meant. I was at a loss. I wanted to confront her, to tell her that obviously she hadn't experienced the pleasure of having a piece of herself cut off and I knew if I said one word to her I would find myself in angry tears. I finally decided that it wasn't the time or place to take my anger out on this naïve member of the female population.

I tried to make redesigning my new work but it just wasn't happening. Nobody wanted to spend money on getting their home to look good when they were planning to sell it, and I was terrible at marketing myself.

Maybe I just didn't believe in myself or in what I was doing.

I began looking through the newspaper for a job so I could move out of our house. I thought that would motivate my husband to complete his never-ending renovations. He was angry because I wanted to split up and I was angry because our house was always in a shambles and because he never talked to me. We didn't have a marriage. To everyone else it looked as if we did, but really, without the communication, we were simply living in the same house together, sharing the mortgage and a piece of paper that labeled him Mr. and me Mrs.

In January 2007 I was hired for an outside sales job. So I moved out. The job was okay, but not as great or wonderful as I thought it might be.

The agony I felt at home, the struggle to stay out of the depression pit, the constant fear, doubt, anger, and sadness, I also felt while away from home and at work. Some days I could hardly breathe. That *ewww* feeling came with me wherever I went.

I listened to positive CDs while I was driving and I tried to keep my mind only on the things I wanted in my life and how I wanted to feel.

I thanked the universe for my healing. Some days were unbearable, though. I felt like I was in another dimension, where nothing I did felt right. Everything felt wrong.

Some days I started crying and I simply could not stop.

# Chapter 34

# COUNSELLOR #2

## Wise Man

Because of the pain I felt in my being and not knowing where else to go to in the hope of finding its cause, I went to see a spiritual teacher who was also a reverend and a counselor. His office was on a houseboat and he reminded me of an old sea captain with sun darkened skin and white hair that was probably blonde when he was a younger man. When he asked me about my childhood, I sighed and told him how I had felt when I was a child and that I had already dealt with psychiatrists, psychologists, you name it. I had moved on from all that. He asked me about specific things that happened at that time in my life and suddenly I remembered that as a child I was going to be the *Princess W ho Never Smiled*, after the fairy tale. It seemed to me that whenever I was happy, I always got into trouble for something so it didn't seem worthwhile to be happy.

It probably wasn't as bad as I remembered because it was a long time ago and maybe I was making more of it now. I tried to brush it off as simply a part of my childhood. He looked intently at me, "Susan, do you know that it was that bad? That is how you felt and it was bad." I felt validated and also a little embarrassed at his supportive manner. Usually I could sense the therapist's neutrality.

I told him about my split with my husband and how we had no communication and I didn't know what to do. I wanted us to go our separate ways in friendship and peace and my husband was so angry he still wouldn't speak to me. I had asked my husband repeatedly about finishing the house and selling it, and had gotten no response for months. I was at a loss; I was angry and simply did not know the answer to our predicament. The counselor asked me if I thought there was a chance my husband would be willing to come and see him. "Probably not," I told him, but I said I would ask. I also told him of the days I simply could not stop crying; that I felt pain in my solar plexus so agonizingly raw, that some days I could hardly breathe.

Every day I filled my mind with positive input, listening to positive CDs, and I imagining how I wanted my life to be. Some days I could almost feel normal. I could almost not feel the gaping wound inside me that kept me in constant pain and torment.

Day after day I struggled with the raw,

unsettling weepiness that overcame me in waves. Sometimes I simply could not keep the tears back any longer, and they spilled over. It was okay when I was alone, and so embarrassing when I was with friends or at my job. I didn't like my new job after all. One morning I was getting ready for work and these words came through my mind: *You have been at this job for eight weeks and already you feel the same as you felt about the job you held for twenty years.*

But I wasn't a quitter! I didn't quit anything I started—I always followed through.

One morning I awoke and consciously decided that I would feel happy, even if that nagging raw feeling was in my stomach. I was determined to feel happy, to think only happy thoughts. If it killed me, I would feel happy.

Later I stopped by the house and I asked my husband if he would finally—the only time in our twenty years together—just this once, tell me how he felt. I begged him. Standing facing the door, with his hand on the doorknob, as he was about to leave the house for the day, he finally said, "I feel lost." I could only stand there in amazement; he had actually said how he felt for the first time in all our years together. My heart filled with compassion for him as he stood facing the door, tears streaming down his face. That lost feeling was precisely how I felt. My entire body relaxed completely and finally I could breathe. I knew in my heart that he was speaking the absolute truth. Relief spread like a soothing calmness through my body and for a moment the pain coming from the gaping wound in my solar plexus relaxed. Tears sprang to my eyes and rolled down my cheeks as my heart opened and with it came the total sadness of our situation. I didn't want to be a part of that way of living, with the constant renovating, the constant upheaval in our home, and the bickering. We only spoke when we argued and I didn't want that. I didn't want to be the one causing him so much hurt and turmoil. I was just as lost as he was, and I didn't know the answer, nor did I know what to do. I asked him if he would be willing to see a counselor who might be able to help him through his part, and surprisingly, he agreed.

We were still at odds as we met at the counselors office. It became clear that we had different points of view regarding our situation and how we came to be in the mess we were in. My point was we didn't communicate. His point was that he was doing the renovations to make our home nicer to please me. Our sessions brought about some insight to our difficulty but didn't resolve the problems.

Another time I saw the counselor, he showed me something out of a book he was reading that related to what I might be going through. He called it 'the dark night of the soul.' It did seem that maybe he was on to something.

The next morning when I awoke, in that split second before becoming fully awake, the words,

*Use the Internet to look up 'dark night of the soul,'* came to my mind.

I got up, made my cup of coffee and sat at the computer. I was surprised at the amount of information on 'dark night of the soul' on the internet. I sat there in front of the computer for hours and cried at the realization that I wasn't alone. I was in this desolate place to grow spiritually, to know consciousness, and I could feel an ounce of relief as I continued to go through my days in utter loneliness, sadness, and despair.

# Chapter 35

# RAGE

## Off the Deep End

Knowing about the dark night of the soul didn't change anything in my life. I felt my life was standing still and that icky feeling was always present. I decided to move back to my house, seeing as I was still responsible for paying the mortgage and the bills. If he didn't want to sell it then he would have to put up with me living there as his roommate. We were by no means back together and my wish was that we would finally realize we could love each other enough to release the other from the bonds of marriage and allow each other the freedom to live as we chose, to go our separate ways in peace, in love, and in friendship.

I also decided to quit my job. I felt relieved when I told my boss "this job is just not for me." It felt right to leave. Even though they didn't want me to go, they were very kind and understanding.

I moved back to our home and resumed my beautiful, insightful walks in the forest and the endured the desolate feeling I felt the rest of the day and night. I was still very annoyed with my husband, especially since he had done nothing to complete the renovations in our home while I had been away for three months. In fact, he had gone to two of his brothers' homes and put down their new hardwood floors! When I found that out, I could only sit and stare at the walls. I was finally pushed over the edge. My mind could not deal with it all; there were no more thoughts left. I could not feel anything and I was absolutely empty. I felt nothing.

Soon after, a huge rage began to erupt like a volcano from my being. I had no control over it anymore. I could not keep the lid on it any longer. One day my husband and I were arguing about the floor that was taking him forever to finish when a huge energy took over my body. I could feel a force from within so great that I didn't know what to do, or how to react. I ended up throwing a bowl of salad across the room, in the direction of my husband. It landed on the plywood floor beside him.

Another time we were having an argument and I told him to stop talking. I could feel him 'pushing my buttons' and I could feel a huge energy coming through my body. The energy seemed to overtake my entire being. It started in my legs and moved up my body and I began to shake violently. My breath came in great heaves

146

and still he kept talking, saying that I was to blame for how the house looked. All of a sudden I saw my two hands grabbing him by his sweatshirt, near the neck, and up eleven plywood stairs we went, I was pulling at him and he was attempting to keep me from harming us both as we stumbled up the steps. The strength I felt was incredible. The power was more than I could control. I thought I was losing my mind. I was screaming at him so loudly I was sure the neighbours could hear us. After that, the rage died down and I ran to the bathroom to cry and wonder what was happening to me. I felt so ashamed. I was out of control and I didn't know what to do. I have never been a violent person, and have never used force against anybody; my explosive behaviour scared me. I could not hold it back—it seemed to have a will of its own.

# Chapter 36

# BIG GIRL, LITTLE GIRL

## Just the Two of Us

My husband has always said it is like there is a big girl and a little girl who live inside me and when the big girl is here, the little girl goes and hides. The big girl is bossy, controlling, demanding, and angry. The little girl is gentle, sad, scared, lonely, and cries. I have always resented it that my husband seemed to be more responsive to me when I cried and felt weak. One time after a rage, I started reading a book, *Soul Retrieval*, by Sandra Ingerman, about what happens when a part of one's soul leaves the body, and I realized that possibly my soul was split. What my husband was saying might be true. I wondered what I needed to do to bring my soul back together. Apparently only a shaman could call the fragmented soul back into the body. Well, I didn't know a shaman. It's not as if they're listed in the yellow pages.

The book I was reading was written by a shaman, so I figured I could learn based on the stories the author was telling. I didn't want to be a big girl and a little girl, I wanted to be whole. As I read, I realized that I could probably figure it out if my husband were willing to help me.

One day I was reading the book and imagining what needed to be done, so I wrote it down. When my husband came home from work that evening, I told him I had figured out what might work. He then proceeded to tell me exactly what I had written. It surprised me because I had just read about it that day and my husband isn't much of a reader, especially about that sort of stuff. I asked him how he knew. His reply was, "Sometimes I don't know I know what I know." I just looked at him in disbelief. We continued on with the plan. I was going to lay on a blanket on the floor, light a candle and have my husband and I imagine the big girl and the little girl integrating as one, coming together in wholeness and balance. He began to explain to me how the big girl scared the little girl so much that the little girl didn't want to come out and play anymore, she was hiding. His gentle tone, understanding and compassion caused tears to stream from under my closed eyelids and the retrieval began. As he gently suggested allowing the little girl to feel safe enough to come out more often, I imagined myself around three years old peeking around a corner in the house and seeing him coming home from work. In my imagination he was about four years old. The realization I received from that first retrieval was that we are all children inside. Our bodies grow up and grow old but in our hearts we are the little girls and boys we were.

# Chapter 37

# SURRENDER

## Where the Ego Dies ...
## And the Soul Lives

In the spring of 2007, my three sisters and I were planning a summer get-together for our parents' fiftieth wedding anniversary. Each of us participated in the preparations for the summertime event.

A disagreement erupted between one of my sisters and me. It had been going on for a few weeks and I was trying my best not to overreact. My explosive outbursts were getting somewhat out of hand. I had thrown many a glass against walls, barely missing my husband's head on one occasion. Always I could feel the force building in my body and I would throw the glass as hard as I could. As the glass shattered against the wall, the rage would subside.

That had to be a better way of releasing rage, or so I thought.

My younger sister lived upcountry from me, so all of our conversations were by telephone (good thing). She said things to me that I thought were very nasty. I didn't want to take my anger out on her—so I really had to work at keeping myself in check. I could feel the anger welling up inside me at her tone and the accusations. I found myself defensive and feeling the need to convince her of my point of view. One time I wanted to end the conversation but she said, "I'm not finished yet." We had already been on the phone for over an hour and frankly, I had had enough. So being nice, I said, "I am going to hang up now," five or six times before finally, gently, hanging up the phone.

I wrote little post-it notes to myself as reminders to stay calm and not fall for her manipulative games, but it was as if she was provoking me. Finally one day I let her have it, screaming at her, trying to make her see my point of view. She wasn't one to back down. I think she thrived on enticing me to the point of anger. I told her exactly what I thought of her and what I had been keeping inside for most of our lives together.

Next came the telephone call from our parents saying how I was wrong and my sister was right. Well, I let them have it, too! I screamed at them. Everything came out about how unfair they were and how they always thought she was right—on and on I screamed. Once I started, I could not stop. I didn't care if they thought I was off my rocker—maybe I was!

Another sister called the following day attempting to fix things. I said what I had to say, calmly defending my point of view one more time, and sure enough it was as though she could not hear what I was saying. So I spoke a whole lot louder! Apparently no one could hear me.

Automatic writing:

*We want to tell you that your dreams are the adjusting of your mind, it creates odd visions. Stay on your path, hold onto your centre. Meditating strengthens this, hold on to what you want. Keep the faith. Remember to remember, stay who you are. Stay inside your body not your head where your ego lives. Your soul lives near your heart. Remember who you really are.*

*Rest your mind, let it go. You are not the one who needs to act out. You are to stay true to yourself, your dreams, your wishes. Keep your mind on what you do want your life to be. Let negative thoughts go into the wind. You shall have much joy. Refocus. Create your world from your heart, dream and wish. Abundance is on the horizon.*

*Be strong in your knowing of what you will learn next. Truth is important in this lesson, you will soon know for sure. Time is of the essence, your life is unfolding in joy and happiness. Live your life in love and joy and more love and joy abound.*

*Move forward with the writing of your book, we will help you, just ask. You will soon see things falling into place; we will be there to help. You may want to feel good, we can help. Begin the first chapter of your life.*

Some days I would just sit and cry, not able to understand what was happening to me. I stopped answering the telephone; I couldn't tolerate listening to anyone speak, especially if they had a long, drawnout story to tell. I felt so utterly alone and frustrated, stressed out and fatigued. I didn't know what to do.

After having fits of rage, I might sit for hours and cry the big ugly cry without the will or the strength to lift my arms to wipe away the tears or the snot dripping from my nose. I could feel myself slipping into the deep, dark pit that I had tried so desperately to stay out of. I could not hold on anymore. I finally stopped the struggle. I stopped the fight. I could not go on that way for another moment. I sat on the sofa, my arms limp at my sides, without the strength or desire to lift them. I sat and stared into space and let myself slip into the deep darkness of that black pit that had threatened to swallow me up my entire life. No more fighting, no more struggle; it was here to take me and finally I surrendered to it.

The heaviness of the silence and blackness pulled me in like a giant net that had captured my being, the darkness devoured me like a ship sinking into the ocean.

The stillness and quiet in the blackness were deafening. It was where true nothingness lived. There was no time, no knowledge, no sound, no light; it filled all space and time, this world of blackness, this land of nothing. I felt like I was floating and drowning at the same time in heavy blackness. Finally, a place to rest and maybe to die, there was such comfort in this place, nothing to do, nothing to say, just … nothing …

Hours would go by as I sat in that state of nothingness. Finally I might have an urgent need to pee and would be brought back to the present. My slipping away for hours at a time went on for days.

Automatic writing:

*We want to tell you to let yourself go. Let yourself be. No rules, no judgment, just you, be who you are, the void you feel is a longing for you. Do what you want today, where is the joy? It is within. Rest. Be.*

*Be kind to yourself today, you hold yourself, you are the judge, you have the choice to feel good or to feel sad, to hold joy in your heart or to drown in your own sadness.*

*You choose. Feel the joy, to create it feel the wealth to create it, you are a wonderful manifester, so manifest. Create your desires. Be kind to yourself and others. Clear the space, let awareness be your ally. Be gentle, do and feel the way you want. The light is seen at the end of the tunnel. Happy thoughts, find them.*

*Go forth with your knowledge and wisdom. We want to tell you to be who you are to yourself; also, you seem to be stalling unbeknownst to us. Your reason is you, so be your reason and move forward, it is up to you to proceed. Move forward now in your wisdom.*

These dark days finally began to fade and I found myself able to clearly feel and know that everything that was happening was somehow completing the long journey out of depression. Instead of constantly paddling away from it, by allowing myself to sit on the bottom of that pit, the darkness left me.

## Chapter 38

# HAPPY FOR NO REASON

## The Secret Garden

I awoke one morning in the summer of 2007 feeling good. I went for my walk in the forest and as my mind began to relax and the beauty surrounded me, I called all my angels to enter my mind and help me make all my dreams and wishes crystal clear. At that moment, a woman loudly called "Angel!" She was calling her dog. It made me smile. I became so thankful for my angels' help and comfort in my life. I could feel the gratitude flowing through my body. I was grateful for absolutely everything—the illness, the long desolate days, the beauty around me, my life, my dog, and my wonderful friends. I was ready to stop judging myself. I could feel joy and move for-ward by remembering my dreams and writing my book as my guides were suggesting.

The good feeling stayed with me more and

more; many days I felt happy for no reason and nothing had changed. I just felt happy for the first time in my life. I felt a sense of inner peace, contentment, and calm.

I had signed up for a psychic development course I heard about over the Internet: Psychic University with Sonia Choquette. I was finally doing only what I wanted to do. If I didn't want to do something, I didn't do it. I began to realize I didn't mind doing many of the things I hadn't liked in the past, even grocery shopping.

I attended a breast cancer support group meeting because I thought I knew why I had healed. Some of the women I had connected with earlier said they wanted to see me more often because they said I was an inspiration. Some said I looked really good. During my time to talk I mentioned that I was writing a book, doing really well, and thought I knew how I had healed. It was because I was able to release the anger inside. I will always remember sitting in that circle, all eyes on me, as one woman asked, "How did you do it?"

Flashbacks of me walking through the forest, praying to the angels to help me release whatever I had to release, drifted through my mind, along with the memory of the rage that had erupted through my body. As I sat there in my chair, my heart sank; I knew I couldn't tell them how I did it. They already thought I was wacko. What was I going to tell them?

I feebly made an attempt to describe how I had

asked to release what I needed to. I said that I was grateful for the illness. One woman stated that she "wasn't quite there yet." So I sat for the rest of the meeting feeling judged by them. I have not been back since. I know some of my dear friends from that group have died. I wished there had been a way for me to share what I had learned.

My sweet mother-in-law passed over around that time and I felt grateful that the time I had spent healing had allowed me to be with her. I sat with my brothers and sisters-in-law at her bedside during the last days as the life quietly left her body. We all knew she loved each one of us, no matter what we had or hadn't done. She had enough love for all of us. I was grateful to have known this gentle woman and to be a member of her family.

Automatic writing:

*We want to tell you, you are on your way, feel good like you do. Be happy you have found your path. Keep the balance; your friends come back because they love you. Follow your truth you will soon see results in your favour, read, learn. Now is the time for you.*

*The awareness you hold within is what lets us in. Keep your mind open to us and others. Learn your lessons well, you are a true teacher, you will find your way, we will be here for you and your book. It is time to begin, you know where to start. Ask for our help we will guide you.*

*We will never steer you wrong, keep going, all is very well. You are very well taken care of now and always. Stay on your path it is the right way.*

*Proceed in your lessons you need the knowledge of the age, choose your teacher and proceed. Now is your time to learn your new skill, to teach and to write of your journeys. Go in faith and love, this is your purpose.*

*It is now your time to learn even more. You have our attention, learn your lessons well. You are on the right path to find your way to a new and happy life. You have traveled a long way to get here. You have greatness within you. You will succeed in this lifetime.*

*To be complete, go within and be complete. Practice being complete, whole, and stop dodging the process with talk talk talk. Feel complete, real, yourself.*

*Relax your mind for some time each day to recall your spirit. You are heading for a new life path, one you have been working on for a long time. You need to discipline your mind. You will. Learn, learn.*

*Train and learn. You are a very important part of this next revolution. You will succeed, you need to teach others.*

*We gather here with you daily to help you write your book, are you ready?*

*We support you in sharing what you know in this issue, you need to tell others. You need to share what you know so others can learn to listen to their inner selves and us so we can help.*

*Dream and wish and manifest, you are becoming a skilled speaker just like you wished so many years ago. Your new skill energizes those around you and causes the focus on themselves, their heart and their lives. Write your story, share your wisdom.*

*To succeed in your business and the world of clarity you must become more aware of exactly what you focus your thoughts on and how you feel about all you think. You are learning the discipline of thought control, you must master this concept.*

*Be who you are, don't hide it. Show people who. Write the whole, everything, you may help many with your book. Your new friends await, begin to share, learn and teach.*

*Share what you know. You know it for that reason. You are a link to some who may want to know. It is imperative you share your knowledge; you all need to know of the other ways to heal yourselves. We are here for you.*

Teaching was apparently to be my new profession. I was to learn my lessons well and share what I was learning, the knowledge of the age, trusting in myself, my intuition and how I was connecting to this knowing, through the writings. Again the concept of keeping my thoughts focused on what I was wanting was reiterated.

# Chapter 39

# MY WORK

## Follow My Heart and Never Look Back

The Psychic University course was scheduled for January of the new year, 2008. I would fly to Chicago to take part in it. I was very much looking forward to it as I have been interested in that sort of thing all my life.

I heard about a cellular healing teleseminar that would take place in the next couple of days. I wanted to know about other ways we were able to heal. When the time came to listen to the teleseminar I was chopping vegetables for the pot of soup I was making so I switched on the speakerphone to listen.

A man began speaking about cellular healing and of a woman who had healed herself from a tumour growing in her uterus without surgery or drugs. I was excited and amazed as he described some of the various things she had gone through. In some instances they were similar to what I had experienced. He spoke about the healing, which was available to everyone, and could be undertaken in a matter of hours through guided processes. I was beside myself in absolute amazement and happiness—I knew in my heart I had found my work!

I signed up for the upcoming workshop and bought the book, *The Journey*, by Brandon Bays. I feverishly read it and could not put it down. Finally I understood what I had just lived through. I realized it had taken me a year and a half to live through what could have been done in a matter of hours through the guided processes. I wanted to know more and waited eagerly for the workshop. I was not disappointed. At the first workshop, I learned how important forgiveness is in our healing process and how to recall, open and release cell memories.

I began to realize, little by little, why I had healed. It was because I was willing to get to the root of the emotions that created this thing they call breast cancer. Even though it was not a pretty sight, releasing the emotional pain, it was where the healing had begun. I didn't know what I was asking for when I prayed so intensely to release what needed releasing. But as ugly as the rage was, it had exited my body. I was so grateful. It all seemed to come to completion when I had let myself rest in the deep, dark pit of the "dark night of the soul," instead of using all my energy to try to stay out of it.

Any doubt about my healing that crept into my mind was relieved at the workshop. I could finally believe, understand, and know that at the soul level I was healed. Most of us are brought up believing only what we are told by doctors. If someone believes that having her breast cut off is the answer to her healing, then that is what she should do. We all have a choice. I have no doubt anymore, and no fear of it coming back. It is finally time for us as women to come together, to stand in our own power and help each other heal instead of having someone cut our breasts off.

I was asked by someone who believed only in conventional medicine if I was in remission. My answer to that question is always the same: "No, I am healed." I can usually see the puzzled expression on their faces. One person wanted to argue: "You mean you are in remission." I stood and in truth and replied, "I am healed."

When more of us *believe* we can actually heal from this thing they call breast cancer, more of us will be able to accept that we *can* heal from it. This will change the consciousness of the disease, bringing women together, allowing us to really feel our emotions, causing the memories to come forth, and finally releasing them, allowing forgiveness to heal.

I believe breast cancer is an emotional disease. It is caused by disconnection from our selves, our true selves, by not living in truth. When we don't love our selves our emotions shut down and that causes our immune system to shut down as well. I don't believe cancer is what "they" say or want us to believe it is. As we shift our belief about what it is, we allow new thoughts and ways of healing to come forth. If what we believe and think about is what we are creating in our lives then we better make sure it is what we want, not what we don't want. That is the Law, the Law of Attraction. Whether we like it or are even aware of it, we have created what we are experiencing in our life. If we don't like it so far, then *now* is the time to change. When this challenge faces us, it is up to each and every one of us to embrace it and take responsibility for our selves and our own healing. There is a way for all of us to reach our inner wisdom to heal our bodies.

Our intuition is important in the process—this may be the beginning of our awakening, our guidance, purpose, and the healing that is inside us all. When we tap into our own wisdom, the healing occurs. This is how it happened for me. Our connection to the divine, no matter what we call it, is our way of walking our path and living our divine purpose. It is an awesome feeling, to live our purpose. We all need to know our purpose, and choose it, and live it.

Our perspective is very important. How we viewed the world when we were younger and how we felt growing up does matter. That is when we began to lock the memories into our cells; as they are opened and released the healing begins.

It is time for us to wake up to this; we have the power to heal our bodies. It is our choice. What we believe *is* important and we can change our beliefs. It is a large part of the healing process. The doubt that kept nagging at me was my mind hanging onto fear. My body was already healed but my mind wouldn't believe it. It is important to address all our parts: our soul, our emotions, the physical body, and mind.

What we think about we create in our lives, and now we have the tools we need to create happiness and joy. Our bodies want to heal. We must be willing to clear out the garbage we are putting into our bodies. Eating what we are meant to eat—natural foods—will help our bodies heal. If sugar and fear feed cancer, then what in the world are we doing to our selves?

To expect someone else to cure us is a mistake in our thinking. Nobody can cure us of anything. We all have the divine power within us; our bodies know how to be and want to be in perfect health and balance. We need to find those willing to show us a new way so we can follow our own paths to bringing our beings back to balance, healing, and wellness. For me it was not using chemotherapy and radiation, but natural, nurturing, healthy, loving treatments. I began to believe my body was healing and the more I believed, the more my mind was able to accept it, and the more I healed to create a beautiful circle of believing, healing and accepting. We are lost until we find our way.

We are emotional beings and that part of us must be honoured. How do we feel about cancer treatment? Do we believe in the mainstream treatments? Why aren't doctors and naturopaths working together to help our body, mind, spirit, and emotions? We are not the cancer, there is more here than just 'the tumour'. We are beginning to understand we need to heal all parts of ourselves; it matters what we eat, we are feeding the cells in our body, it matters what we think. The thoughts we think, whether consciously or unconsciously, are creating our future. Maybe we need to 'check in' and listen with our inner ear to what our thoughts are as we wake up in the morning and before we get out of bed. Are they positive or negative? This is when our mind can be quiet and calm and we may hear what we are telling ourselves. My thoughts used to be negative. I have since worked on changing them, disciplining my mind to remember to love myself, just as I am, including all my faults, to forgive myself every day and to remember all the things I have to be grateful for. These are my new thoughts. They come automatically now, first thing as I awake in the morning.

I have practiced and am still practicing good thoughts, kindness to myself and others and being gentle with myself and others. I use affirmations and mantras to practice keeping my mind positive. We must practice this new way of thinking every day. On the days where I slip and feel the negativity, I know it may be connected to something in the past that can be released. We must release the past. My guides told me that, through my automatic writing, for years until finally one day I caught up. I did the work of releasing many times, over and over until I could forgive the past and everyone in it.

Our bodies have suppressed emotions from a long time ago and possibly from yesterday.

I didn't know how to release this old emotional stuff until I experienced cancer. For me that was my gift. I learned how to release and now I am able to share that know how. We all must let go of our past pain, otherwise we are holding it in our bodies, in our cells. Sometimes we are not aware of what we are holding onto. I knew I felt angry often and thought it had already been dealt with by putting it on a shelf in my mind.

Reality showed me, by having cancer, that I had suppressed emotional experiences and held this anger as a block in my body. It is not always easy to identify and release the past but it must be done. There are many practitioners that have learned therapies like 'The Journey', and many others that can get to the core issue and assist in the clearing out of these past traumas so the body's energy can move through freely.

As we practice releasing, forgiving, thinking and believing, we can heal. Eating healthy foods and doing only the things we love, our lives change.

We don't have to mutilate and poison our bodies anymore. To keep looking for a cure under a microscope is costing all of us millions of dollars and keeping some in devastating, life-threatening fear. The answer is not found in the laboratories; the answers are all within.

I wonder what would happen if money were made available to develop the alternative, complementary, and natural ways, for the practitioners, healers, and leaders of the world who are holding out their hands to help those who believe in another way of healing? How many more of us would grow in our own awareness and achieve this magnificent wisdom and knowledge that all of us have access to? Who knows what would be next—the healing of this beautiful planet Earth?

I don't walk for cancer, run for it, or give money to it and I don't buy breast cancer pink. I already gave a quarter of my breast—I am not giving any more to cancer. I am eternally grateful for this disease they call cancer; it's when my life began, it is the gift. It is a way in which I can relate to thousands of women and men who have gone through the fear and anguish and now can help raise the awareness of our own inner wisdom. This is where the answer is found.

My work, which I love, is reaching out to others who want to heal their bodies and minds, sharing what I know and teaching others another way. This experience they call breast cancer taught me how to live in my body and how to trust my body's wisdom. I learned how to love myself and how to live an authentic life.

I now am an emotional release specialist, having completed The Journey practitioners program. I am an Accredited Journey Practitioner. My work began in this field after attending my very first Journey workshop. Upon returning home my herbalist had one of her clients see me for some emotional issues that were showing up from the client's past. I began practicing the process I had learned from the workshop and sure enough we came to a time in her life when something happened that left her with suppressed feelings that needed to be released before she could be complete. She was my first client and she had many friends she referred me to. I had begun my practicum before I had even been through the program, as I was just learning how to find and release the issues. These first clients were invaluable and I am grateful for the teachings. It was easy for me to get the practice I needed in this field.

Anxiety was a familiar emotion throughout my lifetime. I could always count on it being there. I did not know how life would be without it. A constant mini whirlpool spun in my solar plexus, sometimes spinning out of control to the point of nausea, panic and fear that I always was attempting to stifle or control, usually failing miserably. It never ceased to amaze me that I felt no anxiety when expecting a client or at any time throughout our session. My solar plexus was calm whenever I was doing Journey sessions; my new found work seemed to ground, connect and balance me.

The work itself is a simple powerful process that uses our own body wisdom to guide us to uncover whatever is that is preventing us from living our true life. If we are ill, depressed, or angry, our emotions will help us free ourselves from the past so we don't keep bringing it into the present and future. This is how our old programs keep running, by repeating the same reactions to specific life situations without a way to stop it.

I did not know how to respond any differently until I was shown why I was reacting the way I was. This method has helped me release the past so I am able to live in the present, where life is. This is what I am able to assist others with. When we know how to leave the past in the past and we practice doing that, then we have the freedom to choose our future and more happens the way we wish it to happen, instead of the way it always used to turn out. Sometimes we have no idea of the beliefs we carry and the vows we have made in the past. We need to clear these up and release them from our bodies and energy fields, when they no longer serve us in our life. If we don't know how to release these we must find the help needed. I didn't know how to release the emotional baggage I had carried with me. My guides helped a lot and I knew there was more. I remember wishing I was dead, wishing I could die when I was fourteen, it wasn't until recently when I learned this method that I was able to release my past resentments, perspectives, beliefs and vows. If we have wished we could die when we are young, that wish must be cancelled or, even though even though many years have passed, we are still wishing that wish because we haven't changed it or deleted it. We don't realize the power that is encapsulated in those words. When I had the talk with God after being diagnosed I cancelled that wish by stating, "I want to live!"

It was spoken with conviction, so a new wish was sent out with an intense energy that makes wishes and dreams come true. I also recognized that I had indeed wished to die many years before and now I wanted to change my mind about it. I no longer wanted to die. In telling God that, with conviction, I released the hold my subconscious had on it. Speaking the words aloud helped my conscious mind release the original wish of wanting to die. When we truly realize the power of our thoughts and words we can begin to use that energy to our benefit instead of our destruction.

I had indication of a fragmented soul when my husband recognized there was a 'big girl' and a 'little girl' that resided within me. This can also be seen as an aspect of feminine energy and masculine energy.

When I was in feminine energy I allowed myself to feel vulnerable and was able to surrender, when the masculine energy was strong I portrayed it through anger and aggression. Ideally the best scenario is the balance of masculine and feminine energy within us, a symphony of feminine (being) and masculine (doing). We all have these two energies within and we must use both. When we are in our logical thinking mind we are also in masculine energy, focused, giving, direct, taking action, goal orientated. The feminine energy is gentle, soft, forgiving, receiving, creative and nurturing. It has been surprising for me to discover how many women have overridden or hidden their feminine side because it was not safe and sometimes not acceptable to be feminine while growing up. In more than one session with women we have had to find her feminine self and bring her back. Sometimes she is scared or not trusting of what took place that made her leave in the first place. My experience of different aspects of myself that were not integrated helps me see this in others and this provides an avenue to reconnect those parts of our souls that have become fragmented or divided during trauma. Parts of our soul can be hiding or in some way not in our body because of the trauma. We need our feminine energy and as we bring her back into our beings we realize how we have allowed the masculine way of thinking to rule. We must also find and use our feminine side; our intuition comes from the feminine. It is from this way of thinking and being, not just from the logical mind, the masculine, but from the heart as well. From the inner knowledge and intuition we are balanced in the masculine and feminine and from this balanced state we heal and we will balance this planet Earth as well.

I have also studied and become a practitioner of Emotional Freedom Technique. This method combines modern psychology and ancient Chinese acupressure to rewire our minds. By doing as we have always done in the past without changing these patterns, we have created ruts in our brains and the old patterns and programming run in these ruts. We need to form new grooves. By learning this simple method of tapping on acupressure points we have access to the wiring of our mind and body. We really can change our minds and shift the ways we used to think and believe to form new habits and ways of being.

I conduct talks, workshops, group and private sessions to share and to assist others to experience healing in all areas of our lives, mind, spirit, emotions and body. I use my intuition whether in a session, with a client or living everyday life. My guides are available to me and they always come through and assist.

We have facilitated many fascinating sessions, my guides and me. I am always open to divine guidance; it is available to all of us. We just need to calm our minds to find it and I can show you how. I understand the importance of truth, living from the heart, showing others the way. I love my work! I now have the tools to help others on their healing path. We need to change our minds. Our minds' job is to keep us safe, it does this by judging, doubting and being fearful. It has done a great job until now.

The thoughts we think are a huge factor in our well-being and our dis-ease. Many of us believe our mind is in charge, we have given the job of 'boss' to our mind. If our mind's job is to doubt, judge and fear...then why are we allowing our mind to rule? What will the outcome be if we allow the inner critic to judge everything and everyone? The answer is that we live a fear based existence...which is exactly what many of us are doing right now (as I did in the past). When we hear about someone having cancer, not enough of us truly believe we are able to heal from it. We immediately go into a fear-based attitude. It is this fear-based consciousness we need to change. In order to shift from fear to hope we must practice believing that we can heal. We can practice thinking and believing by listening to experiences of others who have healed. This is how I began to change my own mind about whether I could heal from cancer.

I listened to the healers on *Hayhouse radio.com* every day to help convince myself that I could heal from cancer. They spoke about people who healed from various illnesses. It helped me to believe it could happen for me because it happened for others.

# Chapter 40

# JUST FOLLOWING THE HERD

## Nobody Here But Us Sheeple

Years ago when I worked at the grocery store I noticed customers would begin to line up at the door before it was time to open in the morning and it always reminded me of the milk cows lining up at the barn door at milking time when I lived on a dairy farm as a child. Nobody herded the cows to the door, they lined up on their own; they just knew it was milking time.

It was surprising how many times I could relate the actions of my fellow man to the actions of the cows I fondly watched, raised, and fed. Cows are one of my favorite animals having worked closely with three in particular when I was in a 4-H Beef club as a teenager. They are sweet beings, in my opinion, although not everyone would describe them as such. I can hear my dad's voice in my head saying, "There is nothing dumber than a cow, you can herd them to the open gate and they will break through the fence." Back at the grocery store on more than one occasion, on busy days with line ups at all the checkouts, I would open up another lane and nobody would come over to the newly opened checkout. It was as if everyone was reluctant to move from their spot in the line-up even though I made it perfectly clear my checkout was open. Maybe it was because there was nobody to line up after. We seem to have a reluctance to lead.

I remember being told growing up that I was a leader and I certainly could not see it. For one thing, I didn't have any followers, so how was I a leader? My thinking was that the eldest child in the family was probably the leader; my spot was the third daughter, so I couldn't be a leader. I always did like doing things my way, but I think that everybody prefers that. I was a shy child, teenager, and adult, how could I be a leader?

The day I was diagnosed with cancer is when I stepped into my leadership role because I was not willing to step into the chemotherapy and radiation line ups. That is when I truly broke away from the herd and decided what my own terms were and what I was going to do about the situation I was in, even though I had no idea where to begin and the fear and anxiety were overwhelming. I wonder how many others would rather do other methods to heal cancer but don't know where to begin, like myself. Why don't we consider *all* the possibilities and why don't we have access to them? Wouldn't it be wonderful if all cancer related treatments were available to all of us and not just chemotherapy and radiation? When are we going to stand together and demand that the money we are putting into any part of cancer treatments and research means *all* the treatments not just the pharmaceutical ones? Do we even know where our so called 'funding' and 'donations' are going? I believe the money that is being raised 'for cancer' is lining other people's pockets, because not much is changing.

I attended one of the breast cancer support groups a couple years after I was done with my treatments to prove to them I was still alive and well. As we went around the room I realized that depending how long ago the woman had cancer, the treatments got more radical and severe. It seemed that women with breast cancer of ten years before had had only a lumpectomy and maybe radiation while the women who were newly diagnosed got the whole nine yards; mastectomy, chemotherapy, radiation, and hormone treatments. I brought this observation up when it was my turn to speak (I was getting braver as time went on because they knew I was 'controversial' so I didn't have to pretend I wasn't anymore). One lady said she didn't see it that way and an older lady stat-ed that it was true, she had just had a conversation with her doctor about that very topic.

178

Typical cancer treatments haven't changed in over sixty years! I want the best for my friends, family, and people that I don't even know. I think we humans need to take a stand about this dis-ease they call cancer and we need to change things to be in our favour. How many people have to die because of chemotherapy before we are willing to do something about it? We just keep lining up at the 'milking barn' because we have no other options. Those of us who choose not to do what mainstream tells us to do are apparently 'controversial' that doesn't seem right to me. Why can't we all work together to get this cancer thing into perspective? What if there is nothing special about me? What if the kind of cancer I had does not need chemotherapy, radiation, or hormone treatments? What if there are lots of cancers that don't need the typical treatments we are all lining up for? I wonder what we the public aren't being told about cancer.

I kind of feel like a cow on a rampage! I can feel the passion coming through as I write these words. We must stand together and find new ways to heal from cancer. How many of us truly believe we can heal from this or any other illness? I do! I have done it. If I can do it, and you know that I did, maybe this can help change minds about healing from cancer. We also have tools we can use to help us let go of limiting beliefs and to assist us to believe our bodies are able to heal without poisoning but with enhancing and bringing all aspects of ourselves together into balance.

From the psychic I saw who did automatic writing I was urged to:

*…temper all knowledge with my own. Filter it and decide for myself. Always follow my heart and higher self. If something…even if it comes from someone whom is hugely knowledgeable, if it doesn't sit right then let it go if it doesn't feel right, feel it in the heart…*

It never ceases to amaze me how good it feels to follow through and do what feels right to me. At times in the past I did things because I was told to by those who had authority, whether they were parents, teachers, bosses or doctors. It was something I learned, probably many of us learned and we began to do what those in authority thought we should do. When I was growing up I remember my parents saying *just because someone jumps off a cliff does that mean you would do it too?* But that was the extent of our learning about common sense. Apparently using our common sense doesn't mean using our own minds and feelings to treat our bodies when there is cancer present, but instead to do what those authority figures say we should do even though it involves killing our immune systems with poisons and burning our bodies with radiation. Who thought up these ways of healing? And why do we not check in with ourselves to know if these treatments are okay with us? Wouldn't it be common sense to have access to all that is available to heal from this? Why are we doing things like walking, running and knocking on peoples doors to get money for cancer when all the known methods including alternative and natural remedies are not allowed? Where did our common sense go? We seem so used to doing what we have always done that maybe the time has come to remember to use all our senses to help us decide what is right for us. It is time to have all healing methods included and paid for, not just chemotherapy, radiation and hormone treatments. We need to choose the best ways for our healing. The only way we can choose is to know about all the ways that are available. Maybe then I could trust the system, an all-inclusive system that isn't biased.

When I chose to use my common sense many people thought it was wrong because I wasn't following the ways the authority figures, the doctors, suggested. My common sense tells me we need to know all the facts and truths about cancer, we need to know where all the money is going and we need to know all the ways healing can be achieved. It seems that common sense now-a-days means doing what we have been doing for many years even though it is not working or including *all* the choices available. I choose to use my common sense, wisdom, feelings and make the best choices in all areas of my life every day.

Automatic writing:

*We want to tell you to reap rewards today of sharing the way. Many must be all of who they are and show others how. Be less in the not knowing and stand in your power concerning life. Reap the rewards of standing in the power of confidence. Never let anyone tell you less. Knowledge of truth is time for allowing messages to flow in real time. Follow your heart, teach others how. Live life in freedom and love, assist others in their healing and release of old ways. Delve into the unknown with the inner knowing and truth shall prevail. Love in full range and move forward in this day in alignment with who you are in truth and forthrightness. Allow the timing to be as perfect as it is, feel the flow and let go of the illusion of control. The way will be shown to the completion of the book. Holding on to thought will not access the release. Rest the mind you hold the key to your success, nobody but you. Be free even in this. Practice, stay with an open heart. Listen to the inner calm that is where the answers are. Feel the feeling of the book into reality. Tell your story the way you do and the way you know how. The answers come through in this way the strife and struggle ends and the words begin to flow one after another until the story is done. You will once again find another way to deliver the message. Rest assured it will be done. The passion is here where is the purpose, in the defense or in the delivery? What is the point of the delivery, only to tell your story. Trust.*

My guides' gentle words of encouragement have helped me to keep moving forward in completing this story and to not let fear of what others might think about me stand in the way of my message being carried forth.

# Chapter 41

# MIND BODY SPIRIT AND EMOTIONS

## Us Human Beings

Our spirit or soul lives in Truth. We innately know the difference between right and wrong, we can feel it. Have you ever had a feeling something was going to happen a certain way and it did? The 'gut feeling' most speak about is the soul or intuition guiding that person. Dreams are another way our soul has access to our conscious mind. Years ago I became aware that the things I dreamed about while I was sleeping would come true. These became premonitions I paid attention to. I began to keep track of them by logging them in my journal. Dreams are odd sometimes and they don't always make sense to our logical mind. As we honour them anyway, we may realize how they warn us and guide us on our path, like my dream about perspective. I had no idea how important the concept about perspective was. It is how we see and feel about things. Our point of view about how we thought and experienced life as we grew up has been an interesting concept for me as I realized not every-body agreed with me about what happened and how things were. The emotional release meth-ods I work with have been an important part in my own healing and it has been interesting to know what matters most is how we thought and felt. Doesn't matter if what is remembered was necessarily true, it was the person's percep-tion at the time and that is how it felt and how it comes up for release.

In one of my own sessions I came across the cell memory of what happened during my surgery:

\* \* \*

I was angry at having to have my body mutilat-ed (my thoughts at that time). As I went uncon-scious from the anesthetic the nurses completed preparing me for the surgery. The surgeon cut into my skin covering my right breast. I could hear their conversation; they were speaking about a popular brand of tortilla chip, they named the brand and were laughing and talking amongst themselves about their favorite flavor of these chips. It as if like they were having a chip party right there as they stood over me and were cutting into my body, removing the tumor and having a gay old time. Well! I was beside myself! (Excuse the pun, I couldn't help myself). There I was, lying innocent and vulnerable on that operating table, and there they all were speaking about chips. I was indignant! How dare they get those tortilla chips in my body? It seemed they were getting chip crumbs into my bloodstream as they continued speaking about chips while performing surgery. Why weren't they speaking about healing, full recovery and 'getting it all' (the cancer)? Why weren't they wishing me a good life with no reoccurrence? Obviously they didn't care about me or my situation as they partied on, getting chip crumbs into my veins. No wonder I was so angry about the whole scenario.

I was very angry during my session as I recalled all the feelings and presumed circumstances that transpired during my operation. Even though I was aware of how ridiculous it all seemed, this is what came up: was it true? I don't know and it doesn't matter. I forgave them for being so oblivious and what was important is that by forgiving them I no longer held that contempt in my body or veins. The question that came from that session is: what if it was true? What if that *is* what they were speaking about during my surgery? How powerful are our minds and souls? Oh by the way, one more footnote: before this session I remember seeing a truck with this tortilla chip brand on the side of it. I was on a walk and as I watched it pass by I thought of how much I disliked those chips. Even I, in my perfection and imperfection will eat these chips on occasion. At the time I had no idea why I didn't like the chips.

When I began walking every day I had a few streets to cross before I got to the forest or beach. I could sense my feeling of vulnerability as I walked, the cars were right there whizzing by me. I wasn't accustomed to walking along the road because I usually drove to my destinations. I felt unprotected and a little ill at ease. My opinion about some drivers wasn't very positive at that time. However, when I was driving, I noticed my opinion about the people walking along or crossing the road wasn't very positive either. I found I had this righteous nagging voice inside my head nattering to me about everyone else, no matter what I was doing. As I became more aware of the criticism going on in my mind, I was able to shift it. It was challenging and it did take some time to accomplish the new way of thinking.

I decided to become a more conscious driver; this took a while to finally achieve. After I made the decision I began to realize how many opportunities presented themselves to correct my original critical thinking mindset. I would forget and then it wouldn't even enter my mind to let another vehicle go first. It was all about me first, you can go after me! Several times I remembered after it was too late to let that other person go ahead of me. Then, many times I might remember as I passed the point of letting them in and pretended I didn't see them until finally I could remember to let people go first *before* I blocked the driveway or what have you. It took a while to retrain my brain and not be all about me, me, me. Occasionally I still catch myself, especially if I am in a hurry to get somewhere and I simply remind myself to be more courteous to my fellow human.

I soon began to recognize the pattern, the ways change happens, that repeat themselves over and over again in every aspect of my life.

I was becoming aware of a way I was reacting to what others did and said to me and the idea to change my old ways grew stronger. I realized that my reactions were always the same, the other party was wrong and I was right, and I had to do whatever was necessary to prove it, even if it meant blaming them for the way I was feeling and reacting. This habit made me feel defensive and I often felt that nobody was on my side or could understand how I felt or see my point of view. Then I was overcome by the feeling of aloneness and wanting to get out of that situation to find a 'better' one, whether it was my job or relationship. I thought 'they' were making me feel that way. I realized that this was how I felt no matter who, what, when, where, or how. Simply put, this was my underlying program or pattern that I was living my life through. I decided to do it differently. It was a conscious choice that I was very aware of. I could feel my body tense up when something was done or someone said something that did not suit me. First, I took note of how much it really bothered me, and then I decided to *respond* instead of *react,* which was what I was used to doing. This new concept had its challenges. At first I found myself reacting in the same old way, time and time again, and I remembered only after the incident how I was going to respond and not react.

The second stage was that, as I was reacting, I remembered that I was trying to change this old behavior, but I kept reacting.

The third stage was remembering just before I was about to react and still I reacted in the same old way. Next came the fourth stage; making the choice before reacting and choosing to respond instead of react. This was life changing in many ways. I became more balanced in my thinking and my actions were more in alignment with who I was becoming. My body was less tense. I could feel my mind relax and was more able to think through the process of finding a solution instead of going over what was wrong, or who was wrong and why, over and over, without a solution in sight. I was able to think and act differently than I ever had before. I was remaining calm and instead of the issue escalating, it was resolved either right then and there or a short time after the incident occurred. This took practice and patience with myself and others, I was willing to do my part to have better relationships and to be more understanding of events that happened and not always understand the reasons *why* things happened the way they did. Changing this pattern within myself has helped me to identify it and help others with issues that show up on their path. We usually don't shift completely, all at once, although it can happen. We also need to feel compassion for ourselves as we change the old programs that are running our lives until we become more aware of them. When we decide to clear out the patterns that no longer serve us we must commit to succeeding and use whatever tools and skills we require until we complete our mission. This is where some guidance and coaching can assist us to get to where we want to be and act in concert with who we really are.

We constantly get the answers to our questions, sometimes even before we ask them.

Whatever we just read, or heard someone say, whatever just happened, what we just saw or thought of, are all ways our guides, angels and/ or god/goddess speak to us and offer us messages. When we choose to be aware of this phenomenon life gets better and we get more comfortable with our signs and signals. We can learn to trust these inclinations more than the things people tell us. I trusted the signs and feelings I was receiving constantly, even though my mind doubted and wondered if I was doing what was right and the best for me. I had no way of proving I knew what I was doing, I had nobody to tell me, there were only indicators to go by. I just happened to be willing to pay attention to them and to use them as guidance.

Often the answers are missed and we can't access them because our minds are so busy chatting up a storm, there is simply too much noise. Our souls need quiet time so we can hear; they need space in our Being so we can feel. As we begin to give it our attention we soon become very familiar with it. Our souls are loving and giving and they are meant to guide us, not our minds. As we begin to live our lives through our hearts where our soul resides, our lives change for the better. It may not seem so at first. We don't immediately have answers to why things are happening the way they are, then one day it all comes together like a beautifully woven fabric and the answers are clear, life feels good. Cancer had that effect on me and my life. I felt as though I had been through hell and back and now, as I reflect, it was totally worth every painful step; I decided what I was going to do and what I was *not* by following my intuition, facing my fear, doubt and anxiety, releasing the rage, going *through* depression and making it to the other side, finding happiness, taking responsibility for my health, connecting with my guidance, letting go of my old job, finding my *work*, learning to love myself and living my authentic life.

I would not give up any of the experiences be- cause I would have missed the lessons learned or the great wisdom which came from this adventure. I am in awe as I realize how it evolved into a beautifully wrapped gift, my gift, where gratitude is the end result. Moving in the direction that feels right is the key. Even when others thought it was the wrong way, I learned to follow my intuition, my soul guided me. As we follow our guidance we are lead to our path in life. We become authentic in all ways including the way we speak and the things we do. Do only what feels good to you. Make a list of all the things you can think of that you love to do and start doing them. When I started out I could only think of three things I loved: my dog, my bed and my wine with dinner. I still love those first three I began with and now my list has grown to many: I love to walk, write, read, garden, talk, laugh, work, ski, hike, to name a few. I also love people, animals, birds, nature, books, crystals, sunshine, dandelions, angels and guides, the list goes on. That is the first step in listening to your soul, it is the way the soul speaks to us. Are we listening? Are we willing to do as we are guided? Or do we discount these feelings because we must do what we 'should' or 'have to do'? This is how it all begins. How joyous would life be if we followed our feelings? Can we even consider it? Not yet, then when? What wake-up call will allow us to change our lives? Does it have to be an illness, and does it have to be cancer? We must get off the treadmill    of the old way of thinking and believing. Soon it will no longer sustain us. There will come a day when we must choose either our authentic life lived from the heart and soul or the mundane existence lived from the mind. The day of choosing may come sooner than we think.

What are we feeding our bodies? We all have heard 'we are what we eat', but have we thought that through? Our bodies need nutrition -that is why we eat. We must honour our bodies and that begins with a willingness to start where we are and to get better at learning what foods are essential to our well-being. This may seem easier for some who already have a healthy life-style and who eat healthy foods, but what about everybody else? We need the nutrients; this is what feeds our cells. Cancer cannot thrive in an alkaline environment. Eating dark green leafy vegetables creates an alkaline environment in our bodies. A strong healthy immune system can help overthrow cancer and reduce the side effects of whatever treatments we are taking. We want to nourish our bodies with nutritious foods that do not contain added sugar or chemicals. Food with chemicals feeds cancer by feeding the parasites and candida in the body. Candida grows in the body that is overloaded with yeast and sugar. It creates an imbalance and the body cannot cope with a buildup of candida.

We must stop eating foods that contain yeast, sugar, chemicals, preservatives, additives and stay away from processed milk products. I wondered for many years why we adult humans drink cow's milk. It doesn't make sense to me.

We don't need to drink cow's milk; there are many other ways of getting calcium. We should not eat yogurt sweetened with chemicals like aspartame or sugar. Have you noticed how many grams of sugar are in sweetened yogurt? Too many! This is one of the ways we stay addicted to sugar. We are not aware of how many foods we eat that contain sugar. We must change our diet to natural and organic and eat meat without hormones or steroids. We can eat berries, vegetables, nuts, seeds and zero fat, plain yogurt. Sweeten it with coconut, cocoa, maca, stevia and other natural sweeteners. Legumes and beans should be avoided most of the time according to Loren Cordain, Ph.D, and his book *The Paleo Diet*. We must clean up our diet and stop filling our bellies with garbage that does not sustain healthy bodies. As we become more aware of what we need in terms of health and balance, some of our old bad habits will begin to fall away naturally without too much resistance. There are tools and skills we can learn and practice to help make the transition easy.

How many of us are addicted to sugar? I had a relatively healthy lifestyle and I had an addiction to sugar. That isn't what it was known as, then, it was known as having a 'sweet tooth'. I had a big bad sweet tooth. It owned me. It wasn't until recently that I was able to stop eating sugar. Now I feel light headed and unwell when I eat sugar. I am no longer addicted. One of the tools that helped me to stop eating sugar was Emotional Freedom Technique, which uses modern psychology while tapping on meridian points or acupressure points. I used Emotional Freedom Technique or 'tapping' to help the fierce cravings to pass. I read the ingredients of everything I eat so I am not feeding that addiction any more. I look and feel so much better since I have stopped eating sugar. I drink a lot of water with fresh squeezed lemon juice and take chromium capsules to keep my body healthy and blood sugar levels balanced. Most of us are semi-dehydrated and are not aware of it. I have mentioned to others that most of us go through our days semi-dehydrated but they claim to drink lots of water all day long as they are always with their water bottle. Yet, when they keep track of how much water they actually consume it is not near the required amount needed to keep their bodies properly hydrated. Here is a hint; if you are a large person or overweight you need a lot more water than a smaller body at its ideal weight. We must begin to take responsibility for caring for our bodies and at least start getting enough water every day. If we begin at square one and usually don't drink any water because we are drinking juice and pop, then we have to smarten up and get used to drinking fresh, cool, life-giving water.

Even though we have all heard how fat is not good for us, let me just mention something about this; there are good fats and bad fats and we must consume good fats for a healthy body. I am not going to go into detail because I am not a nutritionist even though I have studied nutrition for many years. However, bananas, avocados, coconut oil, flaxseed oil, and olive oil are good. I have heard flaxseed oil is 'controversial'. I do not know where this controversy came from. If I don't know about something I will investigate and study until I know enough to form my own opinion. I do what feels right or what makes sense to me. A few years back, when margarine was created, we were taught to believe it was better for us than butter. How many of us really believe that? Are we accepting that as truth because our grandparents and parents believed it? We must question where we got some of our beliefs and decide whether we really think that way or if we choose to change our minds and beliefs to be more in alignment with what is right for *us*. We must take care of these bodies; we need them to carry our brain, spirit, and emotions while we are here on Earth.

Our emotions play a hugely important role in our health and well-being. We usually don't realize the programs we are living because of some past incident that happened to us when we were younger. These old ways of thinking and reacting cause us to be out of sync with who we really are. We are meant to be loving and forgiving. If we don't know why we are behaving the way we do and, even if we are aware, how can we change it? That was a major issue for me. The anger I had suppressed in my Being was there but how was I supposed to 'get rid of it'? The answer is a tough one and it lies in forgiveness. How can we forgive something that we are still angry about? I needed help because I did not know the answers nor did I have someone in my life who could help me, even though I had tried for years to get help in this area. We need to release the past. My guides finally stopped reminding me, after repeating it throughout my writings day after day for a couple years, until I could practice leaving the past in the past.

They showed me how I kept the past in the present; I was driving in my car one evening and, as I drove by the street I would have previously turned onto to drive to my home, a wave of homesickness made my solar plexus feel like a swirling pit of emotional turmoil. I missed my former life, so predictable and safe. As I drove I had a vision of the past in the form of a bubble to the left of my head with the words, *this is the past.* As I thought of that predictable and safe past it moved in front of me, near my forehead. The words, *stop thinking about the past,* then *What do you want?* filled it. I remembered I wanted a fulfilling, loving relationship where I was seen and heard, to love my work, to have my book published, and to be the best I could be. All of a sudden the past bubble burst along with the feeling of homesickness and emotional turmoil. I felt my energy surge; my empowerment filled the dream of what I wanted and in that split second I knew I would have all that I wanted as long as I stopped dragging the past into the present. Now I know how to keep the past in the past – I simply don't think about it. Even though this was challenging, I practiced until I could bring my mind to think only about all the things I wanted. When, at times, the past snuck its way into my mind, I practiced my new habit; to make myself feel the way I wanted to feel; happy, content, at peace and connected. I was willing to once again practice mind discipline until my thoughts began to change to what I wanted instead of that old, unwanted feeling of anxiety and stress.

Automatic writing:

*We want to tell you to Be in each moment today and allow the feelings to move through. Keep your mind on moving forward, not on the past. It is good to pause, rest, take a breath. Keep thoughts on the successes you will see in this lifetime. Project forward and use your energy to power the dreams and wishes into manifestations you wish for. Teach others along the way. Soon a new life emerges. Happiness and love are everywhere, feel good and more good feelings follow. Anchor your dreams and follow your heart. Use your power to create as you wish life to be. You have created all you have at this time, now you know how. Create even more of the ways you wish life to be. Focus, dream, and it shall be. You know how. Teach others to dream. Teach others to release, you have an important job at this time. Reach out your hand and bring all into the light. Remember the light is you and* *they are the light also. You will soon see the wonderful results of your time and energy. Success will be evident in all areas you have had your focus on. Look for the joy in this lifetime, it is here. Find your strength and don't look back. Be in the moment of this feeling of not knowing. Then realize you <u>do</u> know. This wisdom of the ages is here for you. Allow it to come through, be the voice for others. Feel good, your work is here. Accept where you are today; allow the feelings to be here. They are a part of the whole. Rest and look to the light for your answers. You are the reason for so much change in this world now. The rest and peace you need is evident. Don't rush, just be in the moment. Enjoy the day as you rest your mind. The mountain to climb is in your midst. Learn to calm your mind and live in a place of peace. You will soon see the evidence of what your work is. Find the space to just be. All is well in our point of view. Trust like you know how.*

Once again my guides remind me to not look back, but to keep my thoughts on what is wanted and wished for. There is power in our thoughts and dreams and we must know that and practice knowing it.

# Chapter 42

# AUTOMATIC WRITING

## Angels, Guides and God

As for my automatic writings, my guides suggested that I needed more discipline in writing my book. They said I needed to get it written to help others. I think they might even have been scolding me about it. It was a slow process. I didn't feel like I knew what I was doing, so I asked my guides and angels to help me. I had a dream wherein I met a woman who had a really long name. She was sitting at a kitchen table smoking a cigarette and she gave me her business card. I told her I couldn't recall her name, and she told me to call her Amy.

The next day I did an automatic writing asking my guides who Amy was. The reply was:

*Well, you asked for a guide to help you write …*

I notice very often as I write this book that I can smell cigarette smoke even though no one is smoking anywhere near me. Sometimes doubt comes into my mind about this book; *who is going to read it?* Once again I trust that I am guided and the audience has already arrived. So I expose myself and all I went through to be here, writing this book. If I help one person realize we have access to all we need right here, right now, I am truly living my life purpose.

I am often asked how to do automatic writing, and this thought goes through my mind:

*I don't know how to tell or teach anyone how to do automatic writing.* And once again here I am attempting to share how I began to write my messages from my guides and angels.

I started by using my left hand and still do. Perhaps I am by-passing my conscious mind by using the hand I don't normally write with. I didn't realize the truth that was coming through at the time. One of the very first writings wrote:

*could you not use sweetner you don't know what sweetner does to you it causes you to become needing too much*

In other words you become addicted to it. That was me. I was already and had been addicted to sugar for most of my life. Almost ten years after that initial message, I have finally figured out a way to get myself off the sugar addiction.

Another writing from then was:

*when you wish for something you shall have it. I heard you wish for a million dollars but you need to feel the wish and teach others to wish for what they want in this life. When you have no more dreams then you die dying isn't bad but you need to live first then when you are here you can live again but you have things to do when you are there. You need to tell everyone you know about the wishing. What is next; you know what you need to do and you don't because you feel unsure but you know so many things that other people need to know but you think they are too scared to hear it. You have to tell them anyway. Don't wish your life away because you need to live it because you know what is next, you will love what is next be happy now for it is coming soon you will see soon enough. See you.*

When I began automatic writing I didn't know how to *feel* the wish before I attained it. It took some time and practice to realize my guides were telling me to pretend I already had what I was wishing for. One of the qualities that assists automatic writing is emotion. It is with the emotion that words print on the paper. I thought I was making it all up, in the beginning, even though I knew I wasn't. Maybe it was the mind's way of trying to deal with phenomena it can't understand. Occasionally I have had to look up words in the dictionary from my automatic writings because I wasn't sure of their meaning and still I thought I was somehow making the writings up. What sense does that make? This is how irrational our mind can be and yet some of us still let our minds rule our lives.

The emotion we need to connect with does not have to be negative; it can be happiness. If I am feel-ing angry while writing, the words print larger than usual and there seems to be more pressure on the paper and still the messages come through, usually soothing gentle messages telling me to *be gentle with yourself and others today.*

Another component is a quiet mind. I notice when I am feeling an emotion such as sadness my mind is in a restful place. When I awake in the morning my mind is also quieter than in the middle or the end of the day.

Trusting the process is another part. When I began automatic writing I was at the point of gentle desperation. I had nowhere else to go to get the answers or help I needed. I didn't trust any one so I found a way to connect to something greater than myself or another. Believing in something greater than ourselves helps us to get out of our heads and allows us to live and connect from the heart. I am willing to trust it, to use it and I have made it my practice. I still use it and write every day.

Automatic writing:

*We want to tell you to free the mind today of thoughtless clutter. Keep it on the intention at hand. Feel the freedom of thought as it manifests itself into the desires you wish for. Use the expression of gratitude for receiving your gifts. Use intention wisely. You are on your path. Let go of the old ways of needing to know how or why. Just let it be and open to the ways of the next that will come to pass. The seeds planted yesterday create today. The seeds planted in this day, this moment are to arrive in due time. Keep the intent on intending. Be hospitable to ideas which come from the ones of unknowing. You shall create and be in touch with masters just as your self. Learn the way for others to hear and use your words. There is profound knowing and knowledge in the times of change. Be aware of the accesses to the ways you wish to know. The key is in your hands to unlock the door to your desires. Look for the keyhole and the mission will be successful. Keep the faith that you will find it and you will. Know there are many helping and guiding you in the midst. Select with care the thought. See the challenge you face and soon you will see the dissipation of it. The curtain or veil persists out of neglect to be clear. Once again step out of society's beliefs, find your joy.*

My guides remind me to keep my mind focused on my dreams and wishes instead of the anxiety and stress that unawareness leads to. What I am thinking about today is creating how I will feel tomorrow.

# Chapter 43

# WHICH WAY SHALL I GO?

## Signs, Signs... Everywhere a sign

One of my clients was writing some notes about her session after we had finished. She asked me if the word she had just written was a correct English word. I had a dictionary in the other room so I retrieved it to look up the word. After confirming to her that she had used the proper word, she then mentioned how she couldn't decide whether she was making the right choice with the changes she was planning on making with her business. I suggested she ask for a sign that would help her ease her mind from any doubt she was experiencing. She could ask for a sign that would tell her whether she was doing what was best for her and her company. I mentioned she might ask for some specific sign or something that she would recognize as a sign to indicate that she was on the right path. She chose something specific, so after giving it some thought she decided that seeing a four leaf clover would be her sign that she was doing what was best. I reminded her that sometimes the signs don't always come in the way we expect them as I opened the front cover of the dictionary we had just used. There lay neatly pressed about fifteen four leaf clovers that I had found over the past few years. I seemed to find them easily wherever I went. After picking the little things I really didn't know what to do with them so I pressed them between waxed paper and gently placed them inside this large hard cover dictionary. I don't know if she believed even after receiving the sign she had asked for if she thought she was doing the right thing. Because our signs and indicators don't usually come in the way we expect them I wonder how many of us keep on doubting.

My friend wanted a sign to know if the writing I just did for her and her family was true and if in fact my guides and angels were communicating with their guides and angels. We were going hiking in the forest the following morning and her sign was going to be finding two feathers. As we were hiking through a forest it seemed to be an easy sign to request. The following day we headed up the trail and came to a big Douglas Fir on the trail that was decorated with all sorts of little knick knacks all crammed into the bark. There were little tokens, charms, ribbons, ornaments, stones and feathers tucked in the bark all over the tree trunk. Maybe that was our sign of the feathers although not very notable, they really didn't stand out in any way and there were more than two feathers. Further down the trail we had forgotten about the feathers, thinking we had already seen them, we were just coming out of the forest, my friend and I, walking side by side talking, when we both walked past twin tiny pure white feathers lying in a muddy patch. We both stopped and looked at each other and began to laugh. That was her sign as plain as day! She picked them both up and gave me one and kept the other as reminders to believe in our guides, angels, and God.

I asked for a sign because I wasn't quite sure at times if I was on the right track as I was delving into the emotional healing teachings. I was using my savings to pay for the workshops and travel to them and my savings were diminishing fast. I just needed some indication that I wasn't going too far off the track so to speak. I was at home one day feeling a little unsure about what I was doing and the direction I was going. I asked out loud to my guides, to the universe, to God to give me one thousand dollars cash in my hands if it was for my best to resume my studies into emotional healing. A few days later I received not one but three thousand dollars.

Signs come in many shapes and sizes. We need to be aware of what the signs mean as we go about living our lives. Sometimes I will see a number, again and again, just as I did in the beginning, with the number 1111. Others have asked me why *they* keep seeing this number wherever they are. Now that I know what it means I am glad to share that it is our opening to possibility, our wishes and dreams, so we must be aware of what we are thinking about because what we are thinking about is what we are creating. Wherever I go it seems I now see the number seventeen. It has been on many license plates of cars or a house address number; I have even seen it on the side of a big truck stopped at a traffic light next to me. I have looked up the meaning of the number in one of Doreen Virtue's books and it basically means I am on the right track. I accept that little reminder and whenever I see the number it makes me smile. I see it often. When we see or hear things repetitively it is usually a sign that something is attempting to get our attention in order to deliver a message. Figuring out the message is up to us. I love the challenge; it can be astonishing and a lot of fun.

I don't know why I found so many four leaf clovers and pressed them into that dictionary we used that day. It could have been coincidental that we just happened to see two pure white feathers on top of the mud while hiking. The money, well, it was an income tax refund and it didn't even match the amount I asked to receive. We can disregard the signs or we can embrace the power of intention and the guidance we are receiving. If we believe in a power greater than ourselves we can believe in possibilities and dreams bigger and better than we can dream for ourselves. We can listen with our inner ear to hear if our mind is disputing possibility or accepting it. Do we believe in signs and magic or do we pooh-pooh it as coincidence? If our mind is controlling what we believe, we need to read-just our thinking and be free to dare to believe in the signs that come into our awareness.

One morning I awoke from a dream about hummingbirds. I got out of bed and went down-stairs to get my cup of coffee and looked out the window to see our automatic sprinkler watering the flowers, shrubs, and grass. My eye caught sight of a hummingbird playing in the beautiful drops of water sparkling in the sunshine. Later that morning I was hanging out the laundry on the clothesline when I heard a very loud buzzing very close to my ear and as I slowly turned my head toward the sound, I saw a hummingbird about ten inches from my head. I must admit a little feeling of fear arose as I wondered if it was planning on sticking its beak into my ear. Later that afternoon as I sat at my computer writing this book yet another hummingbird was buzz-ing outside our French doors. It looked as if it was watching it's reflection in the windows. Up and down the glass door it flew. I was amazed at all these sightings in the same day; I immedi-ately looked up the meaning on the Internet.

Then I asked my guides and angels for some insight through a writing:

*We want to tell you hummingbirds are a sign to*

*you of your wealth, a plenty of abundance in the belief of yourself and your people and your teachings. Your talents and gifts are many. You can see into the inner soul of others. Accept your wisdom for it is so. Share what you know your life expands to teach others. You are of the purpose of this understanding. Teach the way of this small bird, the power of one so tiny is the intensity of the energy in motion. The dream of peace, happiness and abundance of the monetary are evident. Trust. Hummingbirds are for wealth, be the wealth and the healer of all ways, they are all for your undertaking. You also have this gift. Become this angel of healing. This is who you are. Be it.*

I feel joy in my life almost every day. Finally, I know how it feels to be happy. Anger still comes along sometimes, and I welcome it. The rage has burned through. Whatever I am feeling in the moment is what is in the moment. No more eruptions. I am still able to feel anger, grief, sadness, and happiness. All these emotions are a part of me. These emotions are to be felt and allowed to pass through my body and being without suppressing them. That is the point; to feel the emotion, and allow it to be felt. It then passes and soon another is on its way. We are all spiritual beings living a human experience and I welcome all of who I am; my weaknesses, strengths, courage, sadness, and joy.

Another of many writings:

*We want to tell you to pass on this message the hiding of the self is what binds us. To be who we really are is the best blessing. The play is cast. The knowing begins; sharing is where the eternal knowing comes from. Be the sword of truth. Only here will the honour and peace of mind be truly evident. Empowerment is a choice. You choose. It comes with the price of truth. Life has a way of showing the needs of the time. Follow the dreams that you feel. That is why you have access to them.*

*We want to tell you stay in truth. You may imagine what you like. W hat do you want? Stay in the connection a while longer, you will soon see a shift and a knowing will occur. W hat is it in truth, rest here a while the understanding is more important than the actual outcome. The revealing of truth is the nature of the conflict. True freedom comes in the light of forgiveness for the unforgiveable, then peace and healing. You are not responsible for others actions now or ever. You have the choice for freedom of this event. Now is the choice.*

I have learned truth can be a double-edged sword, many are not prepared to live in truth or to hear it. It need not be mean or crass and still at times it bites. We must speak truth and live it.

I am free. Nothing can hold me back from living my whole life. As I step into my life of sharing and teaching I feel a welcoming sense of realizing, deep down, that I knew this all along but somehow just couldn't connect with it. Finally I am here, living truth. I also understand that for some, it may be their exit point, their time to move beyond this earthly experience. For me, I chose to stay a while longer. This is my story, my perspective on how I saw the world and what I went through. It is how I felt and how this body healed. Nobody else's healing will necessarily be the same—we are all different; we all have had different experiences in our lives. Maybe I am among the first to blaze the trail for others. It could be somewhat less intense for those who follow. Not everyone has rage like I had, and if they do, it does not have to be acted out. I have learned through my work that the energy that shook through my body is life-force energy and we can allow it to pass through our bodies without acting on it. There are ways to release these suppressed emotions safely and sanely.

On more than one occasion I have had the honour of helping others identify and release the issues that held them back in life. It is truly amazing how shifting and releasing past resentments can change a person's direction, which puts them on their path where life gets better and the old patterns that weren't working fall away and clarity emerges. From this state of clearer thinking magic happens and opportunities present themselves and as we become more willing to walk through the doors of opportunity, life becomes interesting and worth living. Wisdom comes from the errors in judgment and regrets from the past. Will we choose to feel stuck in guilt and shame or do we choose to learn from our pasts and move forward with greater clarity and wisdom knowing what mistakes to not repeat?

I believe it takes a village to heal. We must

use whoever resonates with us on our healing path. Make the changes in life now, don't wait! "We are not dogmatic;" we use all the resources that are available to us. I am grateful every day for the learning that continues to unfold and for knowing who I am—even if it did cost me a quarter of my beloved breast.

We all hold the key within ourselves to heal our bodies from this they call cancer. It is an emotional dis-ease; there is hope and a way to heal.

And so my life begins …

# About The Author

I feel good about all the choices I made during my time of healing. No regrets. Happiness has opened my being into a trusted and trusting person.

My work as a practitioner of emotional release and cellular healing grows. I love it. I have also begun teaching a class of friends about trusting one's intuition. Through my walks alone in the forest and along the beach I have become even more aware of my guides' presence. As I walk alone, I realize it is an opportune time for them to communicate with me.

Sometimes pen and paper seem so rigid and restricted, compared to a feeling, knowing and/ or concept about something or someone. There is so much insight available. I continue to walk every morning, usually for an hour and a half, along the beach. I use this time to meditate, a walking meditation.

My automatic writings continue as well. When I completed the rough draft of this book, I said to my guides, "OK, here it is, I am finished, now what?" The reply was:

*Show up for your cause. Listen with your heart, you know how. Time is now, your book awaits publication.*

*Don't harness the horse. Let it run free. You will know when it happens.*

Well, that was a good start. What it actually meant took a few months for me to realize, though. Some-one told me e-books were the up-and-coming way to present a book, being mindful of saving our beauti-ful trees. It just felt right. That is how I knew what to do next.

Our beloved Molly has passed on to the other side. I dream about her sometimes and when I walk I occasionally feel her walking at my side. The connection we have still exists; many times I feel she is lying in the back seat of our car, being with me where ever I go just like she did in life. I miss her cute little face and her big brown eyes. She is our little girl, always will be, she taught us about undying love and how to be a best friend to both of us.

Automatic writing the day after she passed:

*We want to tell you Molly is watching you from this side now. She feels happiness and love in her heart. She thanks you and her dad for taking such good care of her. She had forgotten how good it feels to let the body go. Let your heart be glad for her. She will send you signs as she takes care of you from here.*

My husband and I have parted ways; our time together was apparently fulfilled. Whatever karma we held that kept us attached completed itself when the time was right. I am grateful to him for helping me release the rage inside and for all the good times we shared together. He is a loving, giving soul and I am eternally

grateful for his kindness and loving spirit.
Maybe because for so many years I didn't love
myself I couldn't even comprehend someone else
loving me. Our parting has been the most difficult thing I have ever done. In leaving my home
and marriage I have felt lost, many days of sor-
row and fear overwhelmed my being. Our life
together was never bad enough to leave and not
good enough to stay. It seemed we lived in limbo
for a long time. I feel great sadness from the loss,
from the failing of our marriage and many years
together to the desperate ways of trying to make
it work and not succeeding. I don't know what
we could have done to change the outcome. I
can see where things began to go wrong so long
ago. I have learned a great deal since our parting and sometimes I wonder whether if I knew
then what I know now if we might have been
able to turn things around. I do realize that it
takes two to make a relationship work and when
one is willing to change and clear past negative
patterns and programs and the other one isn't
ready it causes us to vibrate at different frequen-
cies and this will ultimately cause a disruption
in the ability to remain together. We must be
willing to work things out at a deeper level and
be open to changing our old ways and habits. I
don't know if I was willing or able at the time
because I was so full of anger and resentment. I
accept full responsibility for my part in the fail-
ure of our marriage. I also feel the gratitude for
all the good times we shared. Forgiveness has

been a powerful healer. I have forgiven myself for not being the best I could be and forgiven him for not being who I wanted him to be and that has freed my conscience from the guilt I have carried. I have decided to learn from my past mistakes and to not repeat them so that guilt is no longer an excuse. We live our separate lives in peace and I feel the love in my heart for him even though we are no longer together.

I have since learned ways to release the past as my guides suggested, also I practice focusing on what I want and how I want to feel. It has been challenging and I am always up for a good challenge. Many Journey and Emotional Freedom Technique sessions later, I have been able to change my old ways. I have decided to feel happy and I practice feeling good by doing the things I love to do. The grief has passed and is passing through, as I write these words the tears roll down my cheeks. I am still allowing the feelings to be felt as I move forward in learning and practicing good thoughts and keeping my mind focused on gratitude and the future I dream about.

My life continues to unfold in wonderful ways. As this chapter ends, another begins. I look forward to all the doors that open and the opportunities that present themselves.

# Afterword

*Fear has taught me to stand in truth and to live my life from the place of truth. Fear has become my best friend; it allowed me to set boundaries when my life was at risk. I learned how to love myself and live in joy—all from my friend called Fear. I took my life in my own hands and became responsible for life here on earth and in accomplishing that I became my own best friend. Fear has taught me to let go of the rope that I was hanging myself by, to expand my dreams because the ones I failed at were just practice runs anyway. My best is yet to be, now that I have befriended this, that I call Fear. I now know how my body speaks to me and I know it never lies. Truth is here in me now and always, I am grateful to Fear my newest best friend.*

*We must become aware of dis-ease in our lives. It need not be cancer! We are able to change now with intention and conviction to do things we love to do and to live in authenticity. We must be the change, we must love, forgive and focus on our dreams. Now is the time.*

*The revealing of the secrets and lies held in our earthly body is the revealing of truth and love. Uncovering the path for others to find their own healing, is why I chose to be among the first. A leader,* a warrior in my own time, a magnificent example of courage to expose the most painful revelations to friends and strangers alike. I stand in truth and show a way to release our burdens; and to find our freedom to love each other in times of war and hatred. I am willing to stand alone and embrace my demons and dragons. This divinity is free for all if only to be willing to lay down our armor and speak from love and truth for others to hear and feel. The connection that is undeniably felt is real, it is the deepest love known. It is creation itself: it is the beauty within and the beauty without. It is everywhere. It is a well-known secret and it is here for all, if only to accept it. The power within is in all, to have the courage to find it is the journey called Life. When we all believe in Heaven on Earth we will all live in Heaven on Earth. It is a reality that lives amongst the illusions that we wrap ourselves in. The choice is ours to live in heaven; we are evidently the followers of this divine wisdom. It is an amazing way to live on Earth at this time.

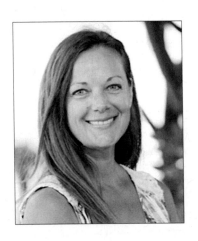

With no roadmap to follow, Susan D'Agostino chose to face breast cancer without chemotherapy, radiation or hormone treatment. Today she is 8 years healthy and works as a professional therapist and counselor. Dedicated to helping others navigate life's challenges and embark on their own healing journey, she makes her home in Vancouver, Canada.

778-846-1211

Susan @ healingeverybody.com